Gastric Sleeve Bariatric Cookbook

Easy and Inexpensive, Excellent Recipes as required After

Bariatric Gastric Surgery, to Optimize your Slimming Process.

Pen name: James Linner

Contents

Introduction

Chapter 1: Understanding Gastric Sleeve Surgery

- **What is Gastric Sleeve Surgery**

Vertical sleeve gastrectomy, also known as the gastric sleeve surgery is a process in which the stomach's capacity to hold the food is reduced by 80 percent. IN other words, a sleeve is created on the side of the stomach, which receives the food in a small amount; the rest is separated through this surgery. This bariatric procedure is also called weight loss surgery as it is used to induce weight loss through a permanent approach. The following diagram shows how the stomach walls are stitched together to create a separate sleeve for food digestion:

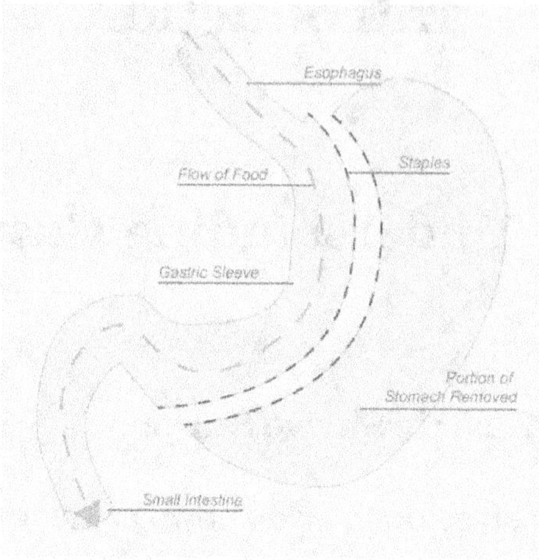

Diagram: Post Gastric Sleeve Surgery Stomach

- **Why is It Needed?**

The gastric sleeve surgery is mainly opted to achieve weight loss. This surgery works for people who are sensitive to dietary changes and just can't lose weight through diet control. So, this surgery finds a permanent solution and reduces the stomach size, which automatically cuts down the food consumption.

This surgery has given effective results, and within one year of the surgery, people should 70 percent weight loss. By controlling obesity, such individuals were also able to resist diabetes, insulin resistance, sleep apnea, hypertension, joints pain, fatty liver disease, and hyperlipidemia. Excessive hunger sensation is also reduced to a minimum after gastric sleeve surgery. The procedure is indeed effective, but it works well only when a person changes his dietary habits after the surgery and follows a gastric sleeve diet.

- **Pre-Surgery Tips**
1. Change your diet and switch to liquid-only diet a week before the surgery.
2. If you are a smoker, then stop smoking at least 2 weeks before the surgery to avoid complications.
3. Discuss your health condition and post-surgery effects with your doctor before the surgery.
4. Clean your kitchen and set up the pantry according to the new lifestyle.

5. Increase the protein intake to prepare the body for quick recovery after the surgery.

- **Post-Surgery Tips:**

1. Switch to the gastric sleeve diet and use more clear liquids right after the surgery.
2. Add protein-based supplements and liquids to the diet to ensure quick recovery and healing of the stomach.
3. Start with the intake of soft food and gradually switch to the proper meals.
4. Stop having heavy, oily food on the table.
5. Light exercises and yoga ensure quick recovery, so try some light exercises 2-3 days after the surgery.
6. Consult your dietician and the doctor after every week to discuss your diet and changing health conditions.

Chapter 2: Gastric Sleeve Diet

- **What to have on the Gastric Sleeve diet?**

It is important to notice here that the gastric sleeve diet plan must be planned according to the post-op healing process. It takes 4 weeks to recover and adjust the body after the gastric sleeve surgery. The food on this diet is, therefore divided according to the five stages:

1. First week: This week is the week of clear liquids only, and the person must only take light liquids like broths, unsweetened juices, decaffeinated drinks, etc.

2. Second Week: In this, a person may start taking food in the form of purees that can be easily digested by the stomach. The dieter can consume:
   o instant breakfast drinks
   o nonfat, sugar-free, pudding
   o shakes made with protein powder
   o thin broth and cream soups
   o unsweetened milk
   o sugar-free, nonfat frozen, ice cream, yogurt and sorbet
   o nonfat plain Greek yogurt
   o fruit juices with no pulp, diluted with water
   o thinned, hot cereal, such as oatmeal or Cream of Wheat

3. Third Week: In this week, a person can start taking proper food but in a soft or semi-solid form, such as follows:

   o   cooked, pureed white fish
   o   soft-scrambled or soft-boiled eggs
   o   silken tofu
   o   soup
   o   cottage cheese
   o   canned fruit in juice
   o   hummus
   o   pureed or mashed avocado
   o   mashed bananas or very ripe mango
   o   plain Greek yogurt

4. Fourth week: by the start of this week, the stomach is almost healed so it can digest food easily. So, the dieter can eat following items easily:

   o   well-cooked chicken and fish
   o   well-cooked vegetables
   o   sweet potatoes
   o   low-fat cheese
   o   fruit
   o   low-sugar cereal

- **What to avoid on a Gastric Sleeve diet?**

Since the stomach size is reduced after the surgery, a person avoids all such things that would occupy the stomach space without providing healthy energy. Following things must be avoided on the gastric sleeve diet:

1. Eating and drinking at the same time.
2. Sugary products and beverages.
3. Alcohol-based drinks.
4. Saturate fats and products containing such fats.
5. Bread, rice, and pasta
6. Highly caffeinated drinks
7. Dry food items
8. Tough meats like beef steak, chops, hot dogs and ham, etc.
9. Anti-inflammatory drugs like ibuprofen, naproxen, and aspirin.

- **What to have on the Gastric Sleeve diet?**

It is important to notice here that the gastric sleeve diet plan must be planned according to the post-op healing process. It takes 4 weeks to recover and adjust the body after the gastric sleeve surgery. The food on this diet is, therefore divided according to the five stages:

5. First week: This week is the week of clear liquids only, and the person must only take light liquids like broths, unsweetened juices, decaffeinated drinks, etc.

6. Second Week: In this, a person may start taking food in the form of purees that can be easily digested by the stomach. The dieter can consume:
   o instant breakfast drinks
   o nonfat, sugar-free, pudding
   o shakes made with protein powder
   o thin broth and cream soups
   o unsweetened milk
   o sugar-free, nonfat frozen, ice cream, yogurt and sorbet
   o nonfat plain Greek yogurt
   o fruit juices with no pulp, diluted with water
   o thinned, hot cereal, such as oatmeal or Cream of Wheat

7. Third Week: In this week, a person can start taking proper food but in a soft or semi-solid form, such as follows:
   o   cooked, pureed white fish
   o   soft-scrambled or soft-boiled eggs
   o   silken tofu
   o   soup
   o   cottage cheese
   o   canned fruit in juice
   o   hummus
   o   pureed or mashed avocado
   o   mashed bananas or very ripe mango
   o   plain Greek yogurt

8. Fourth week: by the start of this week, the stomach is almost healed so it can digest food easily. So, the dieter can eat following items easily:
   o   well-cooked chicken and fish
   o   well-cooked vegetables
   o   sweet potatoes
   o   low-fat cheese
   o   fruit
   o   low-sugar cereal

- **What to avoid on a Gastric Sleeve diet?**

Since the stomach size is reduced after the surgery, a person avoids all such things that would occupy the stomach space without providing healthy energy. Following things must be avoided on the gastric sleeve diet:

10. Eating and drinking at the same time.
11. Sugary products and beverages.
12. Alcohol-based drinks.
13. Saturate fats and products containing such fats.
14. Bread, rice, and pasta
15. Highly caffeinated drinks
16. Dry food items
17. Tough meats like beef steak, chops, hot dogs and ham, etc.
18. Anti-inflammatory drugs like ibuprofen, naproxen, and aspirin.

Chapter 3: The Clear Liquids Diet

A clear liquid diet is recommended on the post-op stage after the gastric sleeve surgery. It is mainly because that few days after the surgery, the healing phase initiates, and the stomach isn't capable of processes nutrients and calories in the food, but the body does need hydration. Clear liquid provides much-needed minerals, metabolites, and moisture that the body needs; therefore, they are given to a person after the surgery for a quick recovery. The following are the clear liquids that must be consumed on the bariatric diet.

1. Broth
2. Unsweetened juice
3. Decaffeinated tea or coffee
4. Milk (skim or 1 percent)
5. Sugar-free gelatine drinks

Gastric Sleeve Diet Recipes

Chapter 4: Breakfast Recipes

Strawberry & Yogurt Smoothie Bowl

Yield: 2 servings

Preparation Time: 15 minutes

Total Time: 15 minutes

Ingredients:

- 2 cups frozen strawberries
- ½ cup unsweetened almond milk
- ¼ cup fat-free plain Greek yogurt
- 1 tablespoon unsweetened whey protein powder
- 3 tablespoons fresh strawberries, hulled and sliced
- 2 tablespoons walnuts, chopped

Instructions:

1. In a blender, add frozen strawberries and pulse for about 1 minute.
2. Add the almond milk, yogurt and protein powder and pulse until desired consistency is achieved.
3. Divide the smoothie mixture into 2 serving bowls evenly.
4. Serve immediately with the topping of strawberry slices and walnuts.

Blueberry & Veggies Smoothie Bowl

Yield: 3 servings

Preparation Time: 15 minutes

Total Time: 15 minutes

Ingredients:

- 1 cup frozen blueberries
- 1½ cups frozen spinach leaves
- ½ cup zucchini, chopped roughly
- ½ cup cauliflower florets, chopped roughly
- 1¼ cups unsweetened almond milk
- 3 tablespoons hemp hearts
- 2 tablespoons almond butter
- 1 teaspoon ground cinnamon
- 1 teaspoon vanilla extract
- 2-3 drops liquid stevia
- 1 banana, peeled and sliced

Instructions:

1. Add all ingredients in a high-speed blender except for banana slices and pulse until smooth.
2. Transfer the mixture into 3 serving bowls evenly.
3. Top with banana slices and serve immediately.

Warm Fruity & Cheese Bowl

Yield: 2 servings

Preparation Time: 15 minutes

Cooking Time: 8 minutes

Total Time: 23 minutes

Ingredients:

- 1 Granny Smith apple, peeled, cored and chopped
- ½ cup frozen unsweetened cherries
- 1 teaspoon pure maple syrup
- 2 tablespoons freshly squeezed lemon juice
- 2-3 tablespoons filtered water
- 1 cup fresh raspberries
- ½ teaspoon fresh orange zest, grated finely
- ½ teaspoon ground cinnamon
- 1 teaspoon vanilla extract
- 1½ cups low-fat cottage cheese
- 3 tablespoons almonds, toasted and chopped

Instructions:

1. In a pan, add the apple, cherries, maple syrup, lemon juice and water and stir to combine.
2. Now, place the pan over medium heat and cook until boiling, stirring occasionally.

3. Add the raspberries, orange zest and spices and stir to combine.
4. Degrease the heat to low and simmer, covered for about 5-8 minutes, stirring occasionally.
5. Remove from the heat and immediately, stir in the vanilla extract.
6. Cover the pan and set aside for about 10 minutes.
7. Uncover the pan and stir the mixture well.
8. Set aside for about 10 minutes.
9. Meanwhile, in a bowl, add the cottage cheese and almonds and mix well.
10. Divide the cheese mixture in 2 serving bowls.
11. Top with warm fruity mixture and serve.

Cheese & Yogurt Bowl

Yield: 2 servings

Preparation Time: 15 minutes

Cooking Time: 8 minutes

Total Time: 23 minutes

Ingredients:

- ½ cup plain fat-free Greek yogurt
- ½ cup low-fat cottage cheese
- 2 teaspoons extra-virgin olive oil
- ¼ teaspoon ground cinnamon
- 2 medium apples, cored and cubed
- ½ cup fresh blackberries
- ½ cup fresh blueberries
- ¼ cup walnuts, chopped

Instructions:

1. In a large bowl, add the yogurt, cheese, oil and cinnamon and mix until well combined.
2. Gently, fold in the apple and berries.
3. Divide the yogurt mixture in 2 serving bowls.
4. Top with walnuts and serve immediately.

Banana Porridge

Yield: 4 servings

Preparation Time: 10 minutes

Total Time: 10 minutes

Ingredients:

- 4 large ripe bananas, peeled, sliced and mashed
- 1 tablespoon almond butter, softened
- ½ teaspoon ground cinnamon
- ¼ cup walnuts, chopped
- ½ cup fresh blueberries

Instructions:

1. In a large bowl, place bananas, almond butter and cinnamon and stir to combine.
2. Top with walnuts and blueberries and serve.

Pumpkin Porridge

Yield: 4 servings

Preparation Time: 10 minutes

Cooking Time: 1 hour

Total Time: 1 hour 10 minutes

Ingredients:

- 1 medium pumpkin, cut in half
- 2 cups unsweetened almond milk
- 1 large banana, peeled and sliced

Instructions:

1. Preheat your oven to350 degrees F.
2. Line a baking sheet with a greased parchment paper.
3. Place the pumpkin n prepared baking sheet, cut side down.
4. Bake for about 1 hour.
5. Remove the baking sheet from oven and set aside to cool slightly.
6. Now, remove the seeds and then scoop out the inner side of pumpkin.
7. Transfer the pumpkin flesh into a bowl and with a fork, mash it completely.
8. Transfer the mashed pumpkin in serving bowls.
9. Pour milk over mashed pumpkin.

10. Top with banana slices and serve.

Overnight Banana Oatmeal

Yield: 3 servings

Preparation Time: 10 minutes

Total Time: 10 minutes

Ingredients:

- 1 cup rolled oats
- 2 bananas, peeled and mashed
- 2 tablespoons chia seeds
- 2 teaspoons matcha green tea
- 1½ cups unsweetened almond milk
- 3 tablespoons almonds, chopped

Instructions:

1. Place all ingredients except almonds in a large bowl and mix until well combined.
2. Cover the bowl and refrigerate overnight.
3. In the morning, remove the bowl from refrigerator.
4. Top with almonds and serve.

Pumpkin & Cottage Cheese Oatmeal

Yield: 1 serving

Preparation Time: 10 minutes

Cooking Time: 2½ minutes

Total Time: 12½ minutes

Ingredients:

- 1/3 cup old fashioned oats
- ½ cup canned sugar-free pumpkin
- 1 teaspoon Truvia baking blend
- 1/8 teaspoon ground cinnamon
- Pinch of ground cloves
- Pinch of ground ginger
- ½ cup no salt added 1% cottage cheese
- 1 tablespoon walnuts, chopped

Instructions:

1. In a microwave-safe bowl, add the oats, pumpkin, Truvia baking blend and spices and stir to combine.
2. Now cook in microwave on High for about 90 seconds, stirring once after 50 seconds.
3. Remove from the microwave and stir in the cottage cheese.
4. Again, microwave on High for about 60 seconds, stirring once after 30 seconds.

5. Remove from the microwave and set aside for about 2
    minutes before eating.

6. Top with walnuts and serve.

Vanilla Crepes

Yield: 4 servings

Preparation Time: 10 minutes

Cooking Time: 8 minutes

Total Time: 18 minutes

Ingredients:

- 2 tablespoons arrowroot powder
- 2 tablespoons almond flour
- ½ teaspoon ground cinnamon
- 4 eggs
- 1 teaspoon vanilla extract
- Olive oil cooking spray

Instructions:

1. In a bowl, add the arrowroot powder, almond flour and cinnamon and mix well.
2. In another bowl, add the eggs and vanilla extract and beat until well combined.
3. Add the egg mixture into the bowl of flour mixture and mix until well combined.
4. Lightly, grease a large non-stick skillet with cooking spray and heat over medium-high heat.
5. Add the desired amount of mixture and tilt the pan to spread in an even and thin layer.

6. Cook for 1 minute or until bottom becomes golden brown.

7. Carefully, flip the side and cook for about 1 minute more or until golden brown.

8. Repeat with the remaining mixture.

9. Serve warm.

Herbed Ginger & Green Chili Crepes

Yield: 8 servings

Preparation Time: 15 minutes

Cooking Time: 8 minutes

Total Time: 23 minutes

Ingredients:

- 1 1/3 cups chickpea flour
- Pinch of salt
- 1/8 teaspoon red chili powder
- Freshly ground black pepper, as required
- ½ teaspoon fresh ginger, grated finely
- ½ cup fresh cilantro leaves, chopped
- ½ cup fresh parsley leaves, chopped
- 1 green chili, seeded and chopped finely
- 1 cup filtered water
- Olive oil cooking spray

Instructions:

1. In a large bowl, add the flour, salt, chili powder and black pepper and mix well.
2. Add the ginger, cilantro and green chili and mix until well combined.
3. Add the water and mix until a smooth mixture forms.
4. Cover the bowl and set aside for about ½-2 hours.

5. Lightly, grease a large non-stick skillet with cooking spray
    and heat over medium-high heat.

6. Add the desired amount of mixture and tilt the pan to
    spread in an even and thin layer.

7. Cook for about 15-20 seconds or until bottom becomes
    golden brown.

8. Carefully, flip the side and cook for about 15-20 seconds
    more or until golden brown.

9. Repeat with the remaining mixture.

10. Serve warm.

Oatmeal & Cottage Cheese Pancakes

Yield: 4 servings

Preparation Time: 15 minutes

Cooking Time: 16 minutes

Total Time: 31 minutes

Ingredients:

- ½ cup low-fat cottage cheese
- ½ cup instant oatmeal
- 2 tablespoons powdered peanuts
- 4 large egg whites
- 1 cup frozen mixed berry blend
- Olive oil cooking spray

Instructions:

1. In a blender, add the cottage cheese, oatmeal, powdered peanuts and egg whites and pulse until smooth. (The mixture should be like a pancake batter).
2. Transfer the mixture into a mixing bowl.
3. Add the mixed berry blend and with a wooden spoon, gently stir to combine.
4. Lightly, grease a large non-stick skillet with the cooking spray and heat over medium heat.
5. Add desired amount of the mixture and with a spoon, spread in an even layer.

6. Cook for 2 minutes or until bottom becomes golden
   brown.
7. Carefully, flip the side and cook for about 2 minutes more
   or until golden brown.
8. Repeat with the remaining mixture.
9. Serve warm.

Oatmeal & Yogurt Pancakes

Yield: 6 servings

Preparation Time: 15 minutes

Cooking Time: 24 minutes

Total Time: 39 minutes

Ingredients:

- ½ cup all-purpose flour
- 1 cup old-fashioned oats
- 2 tablespoons flax seeds
- 1 teaspoon baking soda
- 2 tablespoons agave syrup
- 2 large eggs
- 2 cups plain Greek yogurt
- Olive oil cooking spray

Instructions:

1. In a blender, add the flour, oats, flax seeds and baking soda and pulse until well combined.
2. Transfer the mixture into a large bowl.
3. Add the remaining ingredients except the cooking spray and mix until well combined.
4. Set aside for about 20 minutes before cooking.
5. Lightly, grease a large non-stick skillet with the cooking spray and heat over medium heat.

6. Add ¼ cup of the mixture and with a spoon, spread in an even layer.

7. Cook for about 2 minutes or until bottom becomes golden brown.

8. Carefully, flip the side and cook for about 2 minutes more or until golden brown.

9. Repeat with the remaining mixture.

10. Serve warm.

Protein Ricotta Pancakes

Yield: 4 servings

Preparation Time: 10 minutes

Cooking Time: 20 minutes

Total Time: 30 minutes

Ingredients:

- 4 eggs
- ½ cup low-fat ricotta cheese
- ¼ cup unsweetened vanilla whey protein powder
- ½ teaspoon baking powder
- ¼ teaspoon liquid stevia
- Olive oil cooking spray

Instructions:

1. In a blender, add the eggs, ricotta cheese, protein powder, baking powder and stevia and pulse until well combined.
2. Transfer the mixture into a bowl.
3. Lightly, grease a large non-stick skillet with the cooking spray and heat over medium heat.
4. Add desired amount of the mixture and with a spoon, spread in an even layer.
5. Cook for about 2-3 minutes or until bottom becomes golden brown.

6. Carefully, flip the side and cook for about 1-2 minutes more or until golden brown.

7. Repeat with the remaining mixture.

8. Serve warm.

Chicken & Zucchini Pancakes

Yield: 4 servings

Preparation Time: 15 minutes

Cooking Time: 40 minutes

Total Time: 55 minutes

Ingredients:

- 4 cups zucchinis, shredded and squeezed
- ¼ cup cooked chicken, shredded
- ¼ cup scallion, chopped finely
- 1 egg, beaten
- ¼ cup coconut flour
- Freshly ground black pepper, as required
- Olive oil cooking spray

Instructions:

1. In a bowl, add the zucchini, chicken, scallion, egg, coconut flour and black pepper and mix until well combined.
2. Set aside for about 4-5 minutes.
3. Lightly, grease a large non-stick skillet with the cooking spray and heat over medium heat.
4. Add ¼ cup of the zucchini mixture and with a spoon, spread in an even layer.

5. Cook for about 3-5 minutes or until bottom becomes golden brown.

6. Carefully, flip the side and cook for about 3-5 minutes more or until golden brown.

7. Repeat with the remaining mixture.

8. Serve warm.

Oats & Cottage Cheese Waffles

Yield: 4 servings

Preparation Time: 10 minutes

Cooking Time: 16 minutes

Total Time: 26 minutes

Ingredients:

- Olive oil cooking spray
- 2 cups old fashioned oats
- 2 cups low-fat cottage cheese
- 6 large eggs
- ½ teaspoon vanilla extract
- 4 teaspoons pure maple syrup

Instructions:

1. Preheat the waffle iron and then grease it with cooking spray.
2. In a food processor, add the oats, cottage cheese, eggs and vanilla extract and pulse until smooth.
3. Add ¼ of the mixture in preheated waffle iron and cook for about 3-4 minutes or until waffles become golden brown.
4. Repeat with the remaining mixture.
5. Serve warm with the drizzling of maple syrup.

Sweet Potato & Rosemary Waffles

Yield: 2 servings

Preparation Time: 10 minutes

Cooking Time: 20 minutes

Total Time: 30 minutes

Ingredients:

- Olive oil cooking spray
- 1 medium sweet potato, peeled, grated and squeezed
- ½ teaspoon dried rosemary, crushed
- Pinch of red pepper flakes, crushed
- Freshly ground black pepper, as required

Instructions:

1. Preheat the waffle iron and then grease it with cooking spray.
2. In a large bowl, add all ingredients and mix until well combined.
3. Place half of the mixture in preheated waffle iron.
4. Cook for about 8-10 minutes or until waffles become golden brown.
5. Repeat with the remaining mixture.
6. Serve warm.

Salmon Scramble

Yield: 2 servings

Preparation Time: 10 minutes

Cooking Time: 5 minutes

Total Time: 15 minutes

Ingredients:

- 2 smoked salmon pieces, chopped
- 2 eggs
- 1 egg yolk
- 1 tablespoon fresh dill, chopped finely
- 1/8 teaspoon red pepper flakes, crushed
- Freshly ground black pepper, as required
- 1 teaspoon olive oil

Instructions:

1. In a bowl, add all the ingredients except salmon and oil and beat until well combined.
2. Add the chopped salmon and gently, stir to combine.
3. In a small non-stick frying pan, heat the oil over medium-low heat.
4. Add the egg mixture and cook for about 3-5 minutes or until done completely, stirring continuously.
5. Remove from the heat and serve immediately.

Black Beans Scramble

Yield: 2 servings

Preparation Time: 15 minutes

Cooking Time: 15 minutes

Total Time: 30 minutes

Ingredients:

- 2 teaspoons olive oil
- 5½ ounces canned cannellini beans, drained and rinsed
- 1 shallot, sliced thinly
- 2 eggs, lightly beaten
- Freshly ground black pepper, as required
- 1 tablespoon fresh parsley, chopped

Instructions:

1. Heat olive oil in a non-stick skillet over low heat and the cook the beans and shallot, for about 10 minutes, stirring occasionally.
2. Add the eggs and black pepper and cook for about 3-5 minutes or until done completely, stirring continuously.
3. Remove the scramble from heat and serve immediately with the garnishing of parsley.

Tofu & Veggies Scramble

Yield: 2 servings

Preparation Time: 15 minutes

Cooking Time: 13 minutes

Total Time: 28 minutes

Ingredients:

- 1 teaspoon olive oil
- 1 small garlic clove, minced
- 2 small tomatoes, chopped finely
- ¾ cup fresh mushrooms, chopped
- 1 pound silken tofu, drained, pressed and crumbled
- 1 teaspoon freshly squeezed lemon juice
- Freshly ground black pepper, as required
- 1 tablespoon fresh parsley leaves, chopped finely

Instructions:

1. Heat the oil in a large non-stick skillet over medium heat and sauté the garlic for about 1 minute.
2. Add the tomatoes and mushrooms and cook for about 3-4 minutes, stirring frequently.
3. Add the tofu, lemon juice and black pepper and cook for about 6-8 minutes, stirring frequently.
4. Remove from the heat and serve hot with the garnishing of parsley.

Bell Pepper & Mushroom Omelet

Yield: 5 servings

Preparation Time: 15 minutes

Cooking Time: 25 minutes

Total Time: 40 minutes

Ingredients:

- Olive oil cooking spray
- 6 large eggs
- ½ cup unsweetened almond milk
- ½ of onion, chopped
- ¼ cup red bell pepper, seeded and chopped
- ¼ cup fresh button mushrooms, sliced
- 1 tablespoon chives, minced

Instructions:

1. Preheat your oven to350 degrees F.
2. Lightly, grease a pie dish with cooking spray.
3. In a bowl, add eggs, salt, black pepper and coconut oil and beat until well combined.
4. In another bowl, mix together onion, bell pepper and mushrooms.
5. Transfer the egg mixture in prepared pie dish evenly.
6. Top with vegetable mixture evenly.

7. Sprinkle with chives evenly.

8. Bake for about 20-25 minutes.

Spiced Apple Omelet

Yield: 3 servings

Preparation Time: 10 minutes

Cooking Time: 10 minutes

Total Time: 20 minutes

Ingredients:

- 1 4 teaspoons extra-virgin olive oil, divided
- 2 small green apples, cored and sliced thinly
- ¼ teaspoon ground cinnamon
- Pinch of ground cloves
- Pinch of ground nutmeg
- 4 large eggs
- ¼ teaspoon vanilla extract

Instructions:

1. Heat 1 teaspoon of olive oil in a large non-stick frying pan over medium-low heat.
2. Add apple slices and sprinkle with spices.
3. Cook for about 4-5 minutes, flipping once halfway through.
4. Meanwhile, in a bowl, add the eggs and vanilla extract and beat until fluffy.
5. In the same frying pan, heat the remaining oil.

6. Place the egg mixture over apple slices evenly and cook for about 3-5 minutes or until desired doneness.

7. Carefully, turn the pan over a serving plate and immediately, fold the omelet.

8. Serve immediately.

Mushroom & Kale Frittata

Yield: 6 servings

Preparation Time: 15 minutes

Cooking Time: 30 minutes

Total Time: 45 minutes

Ingredients:

- ½ cup unsweetened almond milk
- 12 large eggs
- ¼ teaspoon red pepper flakes, crushed
- Freshly ground black pepper, as required
- 2 tablespoon olive oil, divided
- 1 small red onion, chopped finely
- 1 cup fresh mushrooms, sliced
- 1 cup fresh kale, tough ribs removed and chopped

Instructions:

1. Preheat your oven to375 degrees F.
2. In a bowl, add almond milk, eggs, red per flakes and black pepper and beat well. Set aside.
3. In an oven-proof skillet, heat 1½ tablespoons of the oil over medium-high heat and sauté the onion for about 3 minutes.

4. Add the mushrooms and cook for about 6-8 minutes, stirring frequently.

5. Add the kale and cook for about 2-3 minutes, stirring occasionally.

6. Transfer the vegetable mixture into a bowl.

7. Now, heat remaining oil in the same skillet over medium-low heat.

8. Add egg mixture and tilt the pan to spread the mixture evenly.

9. Cook for about 5 minutes.

10. Spread the vegetable mixture over cooked egg mixture evenly.

11. Immediately, transfer the skillet into the oven.

12. Bake for about 5 minutes.

13. Remove the skillet of frittata from the oven and carefully invert the frittata onto a plate.

14. Carefully, place the frittata in the skillet, cooked side up.

15. Bake Remove the skillet of frittata from the oven and set aside for about 5 minutes.

16. Cut into 6 equal sized wedges and serve.

Broiled Zucchini Frittata

Yield: 6 servings

Preparation Time: 15 minutes

Cooking Time: 20 minutes

Total Time: 35 minutes

Ingredients:

- 2 tablespoons unsweetened almond milk
- 8 eggs
- Freshly ground black pepper, as required
- 1 tablespoon olive oil
- 1 garlic clove, minced
- 2 medium zucchinis, cut into ¼-inch thick round slices
- ½ cup goat cheese, crumbled

Instructions:

1. Preheat your oven to 350 degrees F.
2. In a bowl, add the almond milk, eggs and black pepper and black pepper and beat well.
3. In an ovenproof skillet, heat the oil over medium heat and sauté the garlic for about 1 minute.
4. Stir in the zucchini and cook for about 5 minutes.
5. Add the egg mixture and stir for about 1 minute.
6. Sprinkle the cheese on top evenly.

7. Immediately, transfer the skillet into the oven and bake for about 12 minutes or until eggs become set.

8. Remove the skillet f frittata from oven and set aside to cool for about 5 minutes.

9. Cut into desired sized wedges and serve.

Chicken & Veggie Quiche

Yield: 4 servings

Preparation Time: 20 minutes

Cooking Time: 20 minutes

Total Time: 40 minutes

Ingredients:

- Olive oil cooking spray
- 6 eggs
- ½ cup unsweetened almond milk
- Freshly ground black pepper, as required
- 1 cup cooked chicken, chopped
- ½ cup fresh baby spinach, chopped
- ½ cup fresh baby kale, chopped
- ¼ cup fresh mushrooms, sliced
- ¼ cup green bell pepper, seeded and chopped
- 1 scallion, chopped
- ¼ cup fresh cilantro, chopped
- 1 tablespoon fresh chives, minced

Instructions:

1. Preheat your oven to 400 degrees F.
2. Lightly grease a pie dish with cooking spray.
3. In a large bowl, add the eggs, almond milk, salt and black pepper and beat well. Set aside.

4. In another bowl, add the chicken, vegetables, scallion and herbs and mix well.

5. Place the chicken mixture in the bottom of prepared pie dish.

6. Place the egg mixture over chicken mixture evenly.

7. Transfer the pie dish into the oven and bake for about 20 minutes or until a toothpick inserted in the center comes out clean.

8. Remove the pie dish from oven and set aside to cool for about 5-10 minutes before slicing.

9. Cut into desired size wedges and serve.

Eggs with Spinach

Yield: 2 servings

Preparation Time: 10 minutes

Cooking Time: 22 minutes

Total Time: 32 minutes

Ingredients:

- Olive oil cooking spray
- 6 cups fresh baby spinach
- 2-3 tablespoons filtered water
- 4 eggs
- Freshly ground black pepper, as required
- 2-3 tablespoons feta cheese, crumbled
- 2 teaspoons fresh chives, minced

Instructions:

1. Preheat your oven to400 degrees F.
2. Lightly, grease 2 small baking dishes with cooking spray.
3. In a large frying pan, add the spinach and water over medium heat and cook for about 3-4 minutes, stirring occasionally.
4. Remove from the heat and drain the excess water completely.
5. Divide the spinach into prepared baking dishes evenly.
6. Carefully, crack 2 eggs in each baking dish over spinach.

7. Sprinkle with black pepper and top with feta cheese evenly.

8. Arrange the baking dishes onto a large cookie sheet.

9. Bake for about 15-18 minutes or until desired doneness of eggs.

10. Remove from the oven and serve hot with the garnishing of chives.

Eggs in Tomato Sauce

Yield: 4 servings

Preparation Time: 15 minutes

Cooking Time: 50 minutes

Total Time: 1 hour 5 minutes

Ingredients:

- 1 tablespoon olive oil
- 4 small yellow onions, sliced
- ½ cup plum tomatoes, chopped finely
- 1 garlic clove, minced
- 4 large eggs
- 3 ounces feta cheese, crumbled
- Freshly ground black pepper, as required
- 2 tablespoons fresh dill, minced

Instructions:

1. In a large cast iron skillet, heat the oil over medium-low heat and stir in the onions, spreading in an even layer.
2. Decrease the heat to low and cook for about 30 minutes, stirring after every 5-10 minutes.
3. Add the sun-dried tomatoes and garlic and cook for about 2-3 minutes, stirring frequently.
4. With the spoon, spread the mixture in an even layer.

5. Carefully, crack the eggs over onion mixture and sprinkle with the feta cheese, and black pepper.

6. Cover the pan tightly and cook for about 10-15 minutes or until desired doneness of the eggs.

7. Serve hot with the garnishing of the dill.

Chicken & Sweet Potato Hash

Yield: 8 servings

Preparation Time: 15 minutes

Cooking Time: 35 minutes

Total Time: 50 minutes

Ingredients:

- 2 tablespoons olive oil, divided
- 1½ pound skinless, boneless chicken breasts, cubed
- 1 medium onion, chopped
- 2 celery stalks, chopped
- 4 garlic cloves, minced
- 1½ tablespoons dried thyme, crushed
- 2 large sweet potatoes, peeled and cubed
- 1 cup low-sodium chicken broth
- 2 tablespoons freshly squeezed lime juice
- 1 cup scallion, chopped
- Freshly ground black pepper, as required

Instructions:

1. Heat 1 tablespoon of the oil in a large non-stick skillet over medium heat and cook the chicken cubes for about 4-5 minutes.
2. With a slotted spoon, transfer the chicken into a bowl.

3. In the same skillet, heat the remaining oil over medium heat and sauté the onion and celery for about 3-4 minutes.

4. Add the garlic and thyme and sauté for about 1 minute.

5. Add the sweet potato and cook for about 8-10 minutes.

6. Add the broth and cook for about 8-10 minutes.

7. Add the cooked chicken, lime juice and scallion and cook for about 5 minutes.

8. Season with black pepper and remove from the heat.

9. Serve hot.

Oat & Blueberry Muffins

Yield: 5 servings

Preparation Time: 15 minutes

Cooking Time: 12 minutes

Total Time: 27 minutes

Ingredients:

- Olive oil cooking spray
- ½ cup rolled oats
- ¼ cup almond flour
- ½ teaspoon baking soda
- 2 tablespoons flaxseeds
- ½ teaspoon ground cinnamon
- Pinch of ground nutmeg
- 1 egg
- ¼ cup almond butter, softened
- 2 tablespoons banana, peeled and sliced
- ½ teaspoon vanilla extract
- ¼ cup fresh blueberries

Instructions:

1. Preheat your oven to375 degrees F.
2. Grease 10 cups of a muffin tin with cooking spray.
3. In a blender, add all the ingredients except the blueberries and pulse until smooth and creamy.

4. Transfer the mixture into a bowl and gently, fold in blueberries.

5. Transfer the mixture into prepared muffin cups evenly.

6. Transfer the muffin tin into the oven and bake for about 10-12 minutes or until a wooden skewer inserted in the center comes out clean.

7. Remove the muffin tin from oven and place onto a wire rack to cool for about 10 minutes.

8. Carefully invert the muffins onto the wire rack to cool completely before serving.

Chicken & Veggie Muffins

Yield: 6 servings

Preparation Time: 15 minutes

Cooking Time: 40 minutes

Total Time: 55 minutes

Ingredients:

- Olive oil cooking spray
- 2 tablespoons olive oil, divided
- 1 small onion, chopped
- 2 small garlic cloves, minced
- ¼ teaspoon dried oregano, crushed
- ¼ teaspoon dried rosemary, crushed
- 1 pound lean ground chicken
- Freshly ground black pepper, as required
- 2 small carrots, peeled and grated
- ½ of medium sweet potato, peeled and grated
- 2 fresh mushrooms, chopped
- 1 small green bell pepper, seeded and chopped
- 8 large eggs, beaten

Instructions:

1. Preheat your oven to 355 degrees F. Lightly, grease a large 12 cups muffin tin with cooking spray.

2. Heat 1 tablespoon of the oil in a large skillet over medium heat and sauté the onion for about 4-5 minutes.

3. Add the garlic and oregano and sauté for about 1 minute more.

4. Add chicken with black pepper and cook for about 5-6 minutes.

5. Transfer the chicken mixture into a bowl.

6. Heat the remaining oil in the same skillet over medium heat and cook the carrots and sweet potato for about 2-3 minutes.

7. Add the mushrooms and bell pepper and cook for about 1 minute.

8. Stir in the black pepper and cook for about 2-3 minutes more.

9. Transfer the vegetable mixture into the bowl with chicken mixture and mix until well combined.

10. Set aside to cool slightly.

11. Add the beaten eggs and stir to combine.

12. Transfer the mixture into prepared muffin cups evenly.

13. Bake for about 15-20 minutes or until a toothpick inserted in the center comes out clean.

14. Remove the muffin tin from oven and place onto a wire rack to cool for about 10 minutes.

15. Carefully invert the muffins onto a serving platter and serve warm.

Tofu & Veggies Muffins

Yield: 6 servings

Preparation Time: 20 minutes

Cooking Time: 30 minutes

Total Time: 50 minutes

Ingredients:

- Olive oil cooking spray
- 1 teaspoon olive oil
- 1½ cups fresh shiitake mushrooms, chopped
- 1 scallion, chopped
- 1 teaspoon garlic, minced
- 1 teaspoon fresh rosemary, minced
- Freshly ground black pepper, as required
- 1 (12.3-ounce) package silken tofu, pressed and drained
- ¼ cup unsweetened almond milk
- 2 tablespoons low-fat Parmesan cheese, grated
- 1 tablespoon arrowroot starch
- ¼ teaspoon extra-virgin olive oil
- ¼ teaspoon ground turmeric

Instructions:

1. Preheat your oven to 375 degrees F.
2. Grease 12 cups of a muffin tin with cooking spray.

3. Heat the oil in a non-stick skillet over medium heat and sauté the scallion and garlic for about 1 minute.

4. Add the mushrooms and sauté for about 5-7 minutes.

5. Stir in the rosemary and black pepper and remove from the heat

6. Set aside to cool slightly.

7. In a food processor, add the tofu and remaining ingredients and pulse until smooth.

8. Transfer the tofu mixture into a large bowl.

9. Fold in the mushroom mixture.

10. Place the mixture into the prepared muffin cups evenly.

11. Bake for about 20-22 minutes or until a toothpick inserted in the center comes out clean.

12. Remove from the oven and place the muffin tin onto a wire rack to cool for about 10 minutes.

13. Carefully, invert the muffins onto a platter and serve warm.

Chapter 5: Lunch Recipes

Quinoa & Veggies Lettuce Wraps

Yield: 4 servings

Preparation Time: 20 minutes

Cooking Time: 10 minutes

Total Time: 30 minutes

Ingredients:

For Filling:

- 1 teaspoon olive oil
- 2 cups fresh shiitake mushrooms, chopped
- 1 cup cooked quinoa
- 1 teaspoon freshly squeezed lime juice
- 1 teaspoon balsamic vinegar
- ¼ cup scallion, chopped
- Freshly ground black pepper, as required

For Sauce:

- 5 ounces silken tofu, drained and pressed
- 1 small garlic clove, chopped
- ¼ cup smooth peanut butter
- 1 teaspoon balsamic vinegar
- Freshly ground black pepper, as required

For Wraps:

- 8 medium butter lettuce leaves
- 1/3 cup cucumber, peeled and julienned
- 1/3 cup carrot, peeled and julienned

Instructions:

1. For filling in a skillet, heat oil over medium heat and cook the mushrooms for about 6-8 minutes.
2. Stir in the quinoa, lime juice and vinegar and cook for about 1 minute.
3. Stir in the scallion and black pepper and immediately, remove from the heat.
4. Set aside to cool.
5. Meanwhile, for sauce: in a food processor, add all the ingredients and pulse until smooth.
6. Arrange the lettuce leaves onto serving plates.
7. Place quinoa filling over each leaf evenly and top with cucumber and carrot.
8. Serve immediately alongside creamy tofu sauce.

Chicken & Strawberry Lettuce Wraps

Yield: 2 servings

Preparation Time: 15 minutes

Total Time: 15 minutes

Ingredients:

- 6 ounces cooked chicken breast, cut into strips
- ½ cup fresh strawberries, hulled and sliced thinly
- 1 English cucumber, sliced thinly
- 1 tablespoon fresh mint leaves, minced
- 4 large lettuce leaves

Instructions:

1. In a large bowl, add all ingredients except lettuce leaves and gently toss to coat well.
2. Place the lettuce leaves onto serving plates.
3. Place the chicken mixture over each lettuce leaf evenly and serve immediately.

Turkey & Black Beans Lettuce Wraps

Yield: 2 servings

Preparation Time: 15 minutes

Cooking Time: 13 minutes

Total Time: 28 minutes

Ingredients:

- 4 ounces lean ground turkey
- ¼ cup white onion, minced
- 2 tablespoons sugar-free tomato sauce
- 1/8 teaspoon ground cumin
- Freshly ground black pepper, as required
- 2 teaspoons extra-virgin olive oil
- 1/3 cup cooked black beans
- 1 cup tomato, chopped
- ¼ cup avocado, peeled, pitted and chopped
- 1 tablespoon fresh cilantro, chopped
- 4 large butternut lettuce leaves

Instructions:

1. In a bowl, add the turkey, onion, tomato sauce, cumin and black pepper and mix until well combined.
2. Heat the oil in a large skillet over medium heat and cook the turkey mixture for about 8-10 minutes.
3. Add the black beans and tomato and stir to combine.

4. Immediately, Decrease the heat to low and cook for about 2-3 minutes.

5. Remove the skillet from the heat and set aside to cool.

6. Arrange the lettuce leaves onto serving plates.

7. Place the turkey mixture over each lettuce leaf evenly and top with avocado pieces.

8. Garnish with cilantro and serve immediately.

Shrimp Lettuce Wraps

Yield: 6 servings

Preparation Time: 20 minutes

Cooking Time: 4 minutes

Total Time: 25 minutes

Ingredients:

For Salsa:

- ½ cup red bell pepper, seeded and chopped finely
- 1 mango, peeled, pitted and chopped
- ¼ cup red onion, chopped finely
- 1 jalapeño pepper, seeded and chopped finely
- ¼ cup fresh cilantro, chopped
- 2 tablespoons freshly squeezed lime juice
- pinch of red pepper flakes, crushed
- pinch of sea salt
- Freshly ground black pepper, as required

For Shrimp Wraps:

- 1 teaspoon extra-virgin olive oil
- 1 garlic clove, minced
- ½ teaspoon ground cumin
- ¼ teaspoon red chili powder
- 2 pounds shrimp, peeled, deveined and chopped
- 2 heads butter lettuce, leaves separated

Instructions:

1. For salsa in a large bowl, add all the ingredients and gently, stir to combine.
2. Cover the bowl and refrigerate until serving.
3. Heat the oil in a large skillet over medium heat and sauté the garlic and spices for about 1 minute.
4. Add in the shrimp and cook for about 2-3 minutes.
5. Remove the skillet from the heat and set aside to cool slightly.
6. Arrange the lettuce leaves onto serving plates.
7. Place the shrimp mixture over lettuce leaves evenly and top with mango salsa.
8. Serve immediately.

Avocado & Tomato Sandwich

Yield: 2 servings

Preparation Time: 10 minutes

Total Time: 10 minutes

Ingredients:

- ¼ cup red onion, sliced thinly
- 1 medium tomato, sliced
- 1 small avocado, peeled, pitted and chopped
- 4 romaine lettuce leaves, chopped
- 4 whole wheat bread slices, toasted
- 2 tablespoons Dijon mustard

Instructions:

1. In a large bowl, add the onion, tomato, avocado and lettuce and mix well.
2. Spread Dijon mustard over each bread slice evenly.
3. Divide avocado mixture over 2 slices evenly.
4. Close with remaining 2 slices.
5. With a knife, cut each sandwich in half diagonally and serve.

Chicken Sandwich

Yield: 4 servings

Preparation Time: 15 minutes

Cooking Time: 16 minutes

Total Time: 31 minutes

Ingredients:

- Olive oil cooking spray
- 1 cup onion, sliced
- 2 garlic cloves, minced
- 8 whole-wheat bread slices
- 1 cup low-fat sharp cheddar cheese, shredded
- 2 cups fresh spinach leaves, torn
- 8 (¼-inch thick) tomato slices
- ½ cup cooked chicken, shredded

Instructions:

1. Grease a non-stick frying pan with cooking spray and heat over medium-low heat.
2. Add in the onion and garlic and cook for about 10 minutes, stirring occasionally.
3. Remove the frying pan from heat and set aside to cool slightly.
4. Arrange 4 bread slices onto a platter.

5. Sprinkle about 2 tablespoons of cheese over each slice evenly.

6. Arrange ½ cup of spinach over each bread slice, followed by 2 tomato slices, 2 tablespoons of onion mixture and 2 tablespoons of chicken.

7. Sprinkle each sandwich with remaining cheese evenly.

8. Cover with remaining 4 bread slices.

9. Grease a non-stick skillet with cooking spray and heat over medium heat.

10. Carefully, place the sandwiches in heated skillet and cook for about 2-3 minutes per side.

11. Carefully, transfer the sandwiches onto serving plates.

12. With a knife, cut each sandwich in half diagonally and serve.

Turkey & Avocado Sandwich

Yield: 2 servings

Preparation Time: 15 minutes

Total Time: 15 minutes

Ingredients:

- ¼ cup avocado, peeled, pitted and mashed
- ½ tablespoon freshly squeezed lime juice
- 4 whole wheat bread slices
- 1 small tomato, cut into slices
- ¼ cup cooked turkey, shredded
- Freshly ground black pepper, as required

Instructions:

1. In a bowl, add the avocado and lime juice and with a fork, mash until smooth.
2. Spread the mashed avocado over each bread slice.
3. Top with tomatoes and turkey and sprinkle with black pepper.
4. Cover with remaining 4 bread slices.
5. With a knife, cut each sandwich in half diagonally and serve.

Tuna & Apple Sandwich

Yield: 3 servings

Preparation Time: 10 minutes

Total Time: 10 minutes

Ingredients:

- 1 (6½-ounce) can water-packed tuna, drained
- 1 Granny Smith apple, peeled, cored and cut into small pieces
- ¼ cup fat-free plain Greek yogurt
- 1 teaspoon mustard
- ½ teaspoon honey
- 6 whole wheat bread slices
- 3 lettuces leaves

Instructions:

1. In a bowl, add the tuna, apple, yogurt, mustard and honey and stir to combine well.
2. Spread about ½ cup of the tuna mix over each of 3 bread slices.
3. Top each sandwich with 1 lettuce leaf.
4. Close with the remaining 3 bread slices.
5. With a knife, cut each sandwich in half diagonally and serve.

Beef Burgers

Yield: 4 servings

Preparation Time: 15 minutes

Cooking Time: 12 minutes

Total Time: 27 minutes

Ingredients:

For Burgers:

- 1 pound lean ground beef
- 1 cup fresh baby spinach leaves, chopped
- ½ of small red onion, chopped
- ¼ cup sun-dried tomatoes, chopped
- 1 organic egg, beaten
- ¼ cup feta cheese, crumbled
- Freshly ground black pepper, as required
- 2 tablespoons olive oil

For Serving:

- 6 cups romaine lettuce, torn

Instructions:

1. For burgers: in a large bowl, add all the ingredients except the oil and mix until well combined.
2. Make 4 equal sized patties from the beef mixture.

3. Heat the oil in a skillet, over medium-high heat and cook the patties for about 5-6 minutes per side or until desired doneness.

4. Divide the lettuce onto serving plates and top each with 1 burger.

5. Serve immediately.

Chicken & Avocado Burgers

Yield: 4 servings

Preparation Time: 15 minutes

Cooking Time: 10 minutes

Total Time: 25 minutes

Ingredients:

- ½ of ripe avocado, peeled, pitted and cut into chunks
- ½ cup low-fat Parmesan cheese, grated
- 1 garlic clove, minced
- Freshly ground black pepper, as required
- 1 pound lean ground chicken
- Olive oil cooking spray
- 6 cups fresh baby greens

Instructions:

1. In a bowl, add the avocado chunks, Parmesan cheese, garlic and black pepper and toss to coat well.
2. Add the ground chicken and gently, stir to combine.
3. Make 4 equal sized patties from the chicken mixture.
4. Grease a grill pan with cooking spray and heat over medium heat.
5. Place the patties into grill pan and cook for about 5 minutes per side.

6. Divide the greens onto serving plates and top each with 1
   burger.
7. Serve immediately.

Turkey, Apple & Veggies Burgers

Yield: 4 servings

Preparation Time: 20 minutes

Cooking Time: 12 minutes

Total Time: 32 minutes

Ingredients:

For Burgers:

- Olive oil cooking spray
- 12 ounces lean ground turkey
- ½ of apple, peeled, cored and grated
- ½ of red bell pepper, seeded and chopped finely
- ¼ cup red onion, minced
- 2 small garlic cloves, minced
- 1 tablespoon fresh ginger, minced
- 2½ tablespoons fresh cilantro, chopped
- 2 tablespoons curry paste
- 1 teaspoon ground cumin
- 1 teaspoon olive oil

For Serving:

- 6 cups fresh baby spinach

Instructions:

1. Preheat the grill to medium heat. Grease the grill grate.

2. For burgers: in a large bowl, add all the ingredients except for oil and mix until well combined.

3. Make 4 equal sized burgers from mixture.

4. Brush the burgers with olive oil evenly.

5. Place the patties onto the grill and cook for about 5-6 minutes per side.

6. Divide the baby spinach onto serving plates and top each with 1 burger.

7. Serve immediately.

Salmon Burgers

Yield: 5 servings

Preparation Time: 15 minutes

Cooking Time: 16 minutes

Total Time: 31 minutes

Ingredients:

For Salmon Burgers:

- 12 ounces canned salmon
- ½ cup onion, minced
- 1 garlic clove, minced
- 2 tablespoons fresh parsley, chopped
- 3 egg yolks
- ½ teaspoon paprika
- Freshly ground black pepper, as required
- 2 tablespoons olive oil

For Serving:

- 8 cups fresh arugula

Instructions:

1. Preheat your oven to350 degrees F.
2. Line a large baking sheet with parchment paper.
3. In a large mixing bowl, add all the ingredients except for oil and mix until well combined.

4. Make 10 equal sized patties from the salmon mixture.

5. Arrange patties onto the prepared baking sheet in a single layer.

6. Bake for about 15 minutes.

7. Now, in a large skillet, heat oil on high heat.

8. Remove salmon burgers from the oven and transfer into skillet.

9. Cook for about 1 minute from both sides.

10. In a bowl, mix together carrot, cabbage, cucumber and scallion.

11. Divide the arugula onto serving plates and top each with 2 burgers.

12. Serve immediately.

Tuna Burgers

Yield: 2 servings

Preparation Time: 15 minutes

Cooking Time: 6 minutes

Total Time: 21 minutes

Ingredients:

- 1 (15-ounce) can water-packed tuna, drained
- ½ of celery stalk, chopped finely
- 1 teaspoon fresh dill, chopped
- 1 teaspoon fresh parsley, chopped
- 2 tablespoons low-fat mayonnaise
- 2 tablespoons walnuts, chopped
- ¼ cup egg whites, beaten
- 1 tablespoon olive oil
- ¼ cup low-fat Cheddar cheese, shredded
- 3 cups fresh baby kale

Instructions:

1. In a bowl, add tuna, celery, herbs, mayonnaise and walnuts and mix until well combined.
2. Make 2 equal sized patties from the tuna mixture.
3. Heat the oil in a frying pan over medium heat and cook the patties for about 2-3 minutes.

4. Carefully, flip the side and place cheese over both patties evenly.

5. Cook for about 2-3 minutes.

6. Divide the kale onto serving plates and top each with 2 burgers.

7. Serve immediately.

Tofu & Oats Burgers

Yield: 8 servings

Preparation Time: 20 minutes

Cooking Time: 10 minutes

Total Time: 30 minutes

Ingredients:

For Burgers:

- 2 eggs
- 2 (16-ounce) packages silken tofu, drained, pressed and crumbled
- 2 cups rolled oats
- 2 celery stalks, minced
- 1 small onion, minced
- 1 tablespoon garlic, minced
- 1 teaspoon chili powder
- 1 teaspoon ground cumin
- 1 tablespoon olive oil

For Serving:

- 12 cups salad greens

Instructions:

1. In a bowl, add the eggs and with a wire whisk, beat until smooth.

2. Add the remaining ingredients except for oil and mix
    until well combined.

3. Make 8 equal sized patties from the mixture.

4. Heat the oil in a large, non-stick skillet over medium heat
    and cook the patties for about 5 minutes per side.

5. Divide the greens onto serving plates and top each with 1
    burger.

6. Serve immediately.

Turkey Meatballs

Yield: 8 servings

Preparation Time: 20 minutes

Cooking Time: 13 minutes

Total Time: 33 minutes

Ingredients:

For Meatballs:

- 1 pound lean ground turkey
- 1 cup cooked black beans, mashed roughly
- 1 small red bell pepper, seeded and chopped finely
- 1 small yellow bell pepper, seeded and chopped finely
- ½ cup fresh parsley, chopped
- Freshly ground black pepper, as required
- 2-3 tablespoons olive oil

For Serving:

- 8 cups lettuce leaves, shredded
- 2 cups cherry tomatoes, halved

Instructions:

1. For meatballs: in a large bowl, add all the ingredients except for oil and mix until well combined.
2. Make equal sized balls from the turkey mixture.

3. In a skillet, heat the oil over medium heat and cook the
    meatballs for about 5-7 minutes or until golden brown
    completely.

4. Cover the skillet and cook for about 5 minutes more.

5. Divide lettuce and cherry tomatoes onto serving plates.

6. Place meatballs onto each plate evenly and serve.

Beef Meatballs with Green Beans

Yield: 6 servings

Preparation Time: 0 minutes

Cooking Time: 0 minutes

Total Time: 0 minutes

Ingredients:

For Meatballs:

- Olive oil cooking spray
- 1 pound lean ground beef
- ¼ cup scallion (white part), chopped
- 2 garlic cloves, minced
- ½ teaspoon ground cumin
- ¼ teaspoon red pepper flakes, crushed
- Pinch of salt
- Freshly ground black pepper, as required

For Green Beans:

- 1½ pounds fresh green beans, trimmed
- 2 tablespoons olive oil

Instructions:

1. Preheat your oven to 400 degrees F.
2. Grease a large baking sheet with cooking spray.

3. For meatballs: in a large bowl, add all the ingredients and mix until well combined.

4. Make desired sized balls from the beef mixture.

5. Arrange the meatballs onto the prepared baking sheet in a single layer.

6. Bake for about 20-25 minutes or until golden brown.

7. Meanwhile, in a large pan of the boiling water, add the green beans and cook for about the green beans well and rinse under cold running water.

8. With a paper towel pat dry the beans completely.

9. Transfer the beans into a large salad bowl and drizzle with oil.

10. Divide the meatballs onto serving plates and serve alongside the green beans

Beef Koftas with Yogurt Sauce

Yield: 6 servings

Preparation Time: 15 minutes

Cooking Time: 10 minutes

Total Time: 25 minutes

Ingredients:

For Beef Koftas:

- 1 pound lean ground beef
- 2 tablespoons fat-free plain Greek yogurt
- 2 tablespoons yellow onion, grated
- 2 teaspoons garlic, minced
- 2 tablespoons fresh cilantro, minced
- 1 teaspoon ground coriander
- 1 teaspoon ground cumin
- ½ teaspoon ground turmeric
- Salt and freshly ground black pepper, as required
- 1 tablespoon olive oil

For Yogurt Sauce:

- ½ cup fat-free plain Greek yogurt
- ¼ cup cucumber, peeled, seeded and chopped finely
- 2 teaspoons garlic, minced
- 1 teaspoon ground coriander

- 1 teaspoon ground cumin

- ½ teaspoon red pepper flakes, crushed

Instructions:

1. For koftas: in a large bowl, add all the ingredients except for oil and mix until well combined.

2. Make 12 equal sized oblong patties from the mixture.

3. Heat the oil in a large non-stick skillet over medium-high heat and cook the patties for 10 minutes or until browned from both sides, flipping occasionally.

4. Meanwhile, for sauce: in a bowl, add all the ingredients and mix until well combined.

5. Serve the Koftas with the yogurt sauce.

Chicken Stuffed Avocados

Yield: 4 servings

Preparation Time: 15 minutes

Total Time: 15 minutes

Ingredients:

- 1 large avocado, halved and pitted
- 2 tablespoons freshly squeezed lime juice
- 2 cup cooked chicken, shredded
- ¼ cup red onion, chopped finely
- 1/3 cup fat-free plain Greek yogurt
- 1 teaspoon Dijon mustard
- Pinch of cayenne pepper
- Freshly ground black pepper, as required
- 2 tablespoon fresh cilantro, minced

Instructions:

1. Carefully, scoop out the flesh from middle of each avocado half.
2. In a bowl, add the scooped out avocado flesh and lime juice and with a fork, mash until well combined.
3. Add the remaining ingredients and stir to combine.
4. Divide the chicken mixture into avocado halves evenly.
5. Serve immediately.

Turkey Stuffed Zucchini

Yield: 8 servings

Preparation Time: 20 minutes

Cooking Time: 31 minutes

Total Time: 51 minutes

Ingredients:

- 4 medium zucchinis
- 1 pound lean ground turkey breast
- ½ cup white onion, chopped
- ½ pound fresh mushrooms, sliced
- 1 large tomato, chopped
- 1 egg, beaten
- ¾ cup sugar-free spaghetti sauce
- ¼ cup seasoned whole wheat bread crumbs
- Freshly ground black pepper, as required
- 1 cup low-fat mozzarella cheese, shredded

Instructions:

1. Preheat your oven to350 degrees F.
2. Cut each zucchini in half lengthwise.
3. With a knife, cut a thin slice from the bottom of each zucchini to allow zucchini to sit flat.

4. With a small spoon, scoop out the pulp from each zucchini half, leaving ¼-inch shells.

5. Transfer the zucchini pulp into a large bowl and set aside.

6. Arrange the zucchini shells into an ungreased microwave-safe baking dish.

7. Cover the baking dish and microwave on High for about 3 minutes.

8. Drain the water from microwave and set aside.

9. Heat a large non-stick wok over medium heat and cook the ground turkey and onion for about 6-8 minutes or until meat is no longer pink; drain.

10. Remove from the heat.

11. In the bowl of zucchini pulp, add the cooked turkey, mushrooms, tomato, egg, spaghetti sauce, black pepper and ½ cup of the cheese and mix until well combined.

12. Place about ¼ cup of the turkey mixture into each zucchini shell and sprinkle with the remaining cheese.

13. Bake for about 20 minutes or until top becomes golden brown.

Veggies Stuffed Zucchini

Yield: 8 servings

Preparation Time: 20 minutes

Cooking Time: 18 minutes

Total Time: 38 minutes

Ingredients:

- Olive oil cooking spray
- 4 medium zucchinis, halved lengthwise
- 1 cup red bell pepper, seeded and minced
- ½ cup Kalamata olives, pitted and minced
- ½ cup fresh tomatoes, minced
- 1 teaspoon garlic, minced
- 1 tablespoon dried oregano, crushed
- Freshly ground black pepper, as required
- ½ cup feta cheese, crumbled

Instructions:

1. Preheat your oven to350 degrees F.
2. Grease a large baking sheet with cooking spray.
3. With a melon baller, scoop out the flesh of each zucchini half.
4. In a bowl, add the bell pepper, olives, tomatoes, garlic, oregano and black pepper and mix well.
5. Stuff each zucchini half with the veggie mixture evenly.

6. Arrange the zucchini halves onto the prepared baking sheet and bake for about 15 minutes.

7. Now, set the oven to broiler on high.

8. Top each zucchini half with feta cheese and broil for about 3 minutes.

9. Serve hot.

Stuffed Bell Peppers

Yield: 4 servings

Preparation Time: 20 minutes

Cooking Time: 40 minutes

Total Time: 1 hour

Ingredients:

- 2 garlic cloves, minced
- 2 teaspoons fresh lemon zest, grated finely
- 2 teaspoons fresh thyme, minced
- 1 teaspoon ground cumin
- ½ teaspoon cayenne pepper
- ¼ teaspoon red pepper flakes, crushed
- 3 teaspoons olive oil, divided
- 2 tablespoons freshly squeezed lemon juice
- 14 ounces skinless, boneless chicken breasts, cut into thin strips
- 4 large green bell peppers
- 1 large onion, sliced
- ¾ cup cherry tomatoes, sliced
- 1 cup canned black beans, rinsed and drained

Instructions:

1. In a large bowl, add the garlic, lemon zest, thyme, spices, 1bteaspoon of oil and lemon juice and mix until well combined.

2. Add the chicken strips and coat with marinade generously. Cover and refrigerate to marinate for about 2 hours.

3. Preheat your oven to400 degrees F.

4. Line a roasting pan with a piece of foil.

5. Arrange the bell peppers into prepared roasting pan.

6. Roast for about 15-20 minutes, flipping occasionally.

7. Remove the bell peppers from oven and immediately, transfer into a paper bag.

8. Seal the top of paper bag by rolling it closed tightly. Set aside for at least 10 minutes.

9. Remove the bell peppers from bag.

10. With a knife, carefully, slice the top.

11. Carefully, peel off the skin of each bell pepper and discard the seeds and pith. Set aside.

12. For stuffing mixture: in a large skillet, heat remaining oil over medium-high heat.

13. Add the onion and sauté for about 8-10 minutes. Transfer the onion into a bowl.

14. In the same skillet, add the chicken and cook for about 8 minutes.

15. Stir in the tomatoes, beans and cooked onion and cook for about 1-2 minutes and remove from heat.

16. Meanwhile for sauce: in a bowl, add yogurt, avocado and lime juice and with a stick blender, blend well.

17. Add in the cilantro and gently, stir to combine.

18. Arrange the bell peppers onto serving plates.

19. Stuff the bell peppers with chicken mixture evenly and serve alongside the yogurt sauce.

Stuffed Acorn Squash

Yield: 4 servings

Preparation Time: 20 minutes

Cooking Time: 50 minutes

Total Time: 1 hour 10 minutes

Ingredients:

- 2 acorn squash, halved and seeded
- 1 pound lean ground turkey breast
- 1 cup red onion, chopped
- 1 cup celery stalk, chopped
- 1 cup fresh button mushrooms, sliced
- 8 ounces sugar-free tomato sauce
- 1 teaspoon dried oregano, crushed
- 1 teaspoon dried basil, crushed
- Freshly ground black pepper, as required
- 1 cup low-fat Cheddar cheese, shredded

Instructions:

1. Preheat your oven to350 degrees F.
2. In the bottom of a microwave-safe glass baking dish, arrange the squash halves, cut side down.
3. Microwave on High for about 20 minutes or until almost tender.

4. Heat a large non-stick wok over medium heat and cook the ground turkey for about 4-5 minutes or until meat is browned.

5. Drain the grease.

6. Add the onion and celery and cook for about 3-4 minutes.

7. Add in the mushrooms and cook for about 2-3 minutes more.

8. Stir in the tomato sauce, dried herbs and black pepper and remove from the heat.

9. Spoon the turkey mixture into each squash half.

10. Cover the baking dish and bake for about 15 minutes.

11. Uncover the baking dish and sprinkle each squash half with Cheddar cheese.

12. Bake, uncovered for about 3-5 minutes or until the cheese becomes bubbly.

13. Serve hot.

Beef Kabobs

Yield: 6 servings

Preparation Time: 15 minutes

Cooking Time: 8 minutes

Total Time: 23 minutes

Ingredients:

- 3 garlic cloves, minced
- 1 tablespoon fresh lemon zest, grated
- 2 teaspoons fresh rosemary, minced
- 2 teaspoons fresh parsley, minced
- 2 teaspoons fresh oregano, minced
- 2 teaspoons fresh thyme, minced
- 4 tablespoons olive oil
- 2 tablespoons freshly squeezed lemon juice
- Salt and freshly ground black pepper, as required
- 2 pounds beef sirloin, cut into cubes
- Olive oil cooking spray

Instructions:

1. In a bowl, add all the ingredients except the beef and cooking spray and mix well.
2. Add the beef and coat with the herb mixture generously.
3. Refrigerate to marinate for at least 20-30 minutes.

4. Preheat the grill to medium-high heat. Grease the grill grate.

5. Remove the beef cubes from the marinade and thread onto the metal skewers.

6. Place the skewers onto the grill and cook for about 6-8 minutes, flipping after every 2 minutes.

7. Remove from the grill and place onto a platter for about 5 minutes before serving.

Chicken & Broccoli Kabobs

Yield: 6 servings

Preparation Time: 15 minutes

Cooking Time: 20 minutes

Total Time: 35 minutes

Ingredients:

- 1½ pounds skinless, boneless chicken breasts, cubed
- 2 tablespoons olive oil, divided
- 2 tablespoons dried marjoram, crushed
- 2 garlic cloves, minced
- 2 tablespoons tomato paste
- 4 cups broccoli florets
- Freshly ground black pepper, as required

Instructions:

1. In a bowl, add the chicken, 1 tablespoon of oil, marjoram, garlic, tomato paste, broccoli and black pepper and mix well.
2. Cover the bowl and set aside at room temperature for about 10-15 minutes.
3. Thread the chicken and broccoli onto pre-soaked wooden skewers.

4. In a large grill pan, heat remaining oil over medium heat and cook chicken skewers and cook for about 9-10 minutes per side or until desired doneness.
5. Serve hot.

Parsley Shrimp

Yield: 3 servings

Preparation Time: 15 minutes

Cooking Time: 7 minutes

Total Time: 23 minutes

Ingredients:

* 2 tablespoons olive oil
* 1 pound medium shrimp, peeled and deveined
* 3 garlic cloves, minced
* 1 lemon, sliced thinly
* ½ teaspoon red pepper flakes, crushed
* Salt, as required
* 2 tablespoons water
* 1 tablespoon freshly squeezed lemon juice
* 2 tablespoons fresh parsley, chopped

Instructions:

1. Heat the oil in a large skillet over medium heat and cook oil the shrimp, garlic, lemon slices, red pepper flakes and salt for about 3 minutes per side, stirring occasionally.
2. Stir in the water, lemon juice and parsley and immediately, remove from the heat.
3. Serve hot.

Garlicky Shrimp

Yield: 2 servings

Preparation Time: 15 minutes

Cooking Time: 7 minutes

Total Time: 22 minutes

Ingredients:

- 1 tablespoon olive oil
- 1 scallion, chopped
- 3 garlic cloves, minced
- ¼ teaspoon fresh ginger, minced
- ¾ pound shrimp, peeled and deveined
- 1 tablespoon fresh lemon juice
- Salt and freshly ground black pepper, as required

Instructions:

1. Heat the oil in a large skillet over medium heat and sauté the scallion for about 1-2 minutes.
2. Add the garlic and ginger and sauté for about 1 minute.
3. Add the shrimp, lemon juice, salt and black pepper and cook for about 3-4 minutes or until done completely.
4. Serve hot.

Cod & Veggie Pizza

Yield: 3 servings

Preparation Time: 20 minutes

Cooking Time: 1 hour

Total Time: 1 hour 20 minutes

Ingredients:

For Base:

- Olive oil cooking spray
- ¼ cup oat flour
- 2 teaspoons dried rosemary, crushed
- Freshly ground black pepper, as required
- 4 egg whites
- 2½ teaspoons olive oil
- ½ cup low-fat Parmesan cheese, grated freshly
- 2 cups zucchini, grated and squeezed

For Topping:

- 1 cup tomato paste
- 1 teaspoon fresh rosemary, minced
- 1 teaspoon fresh basil, minced
- Freshly ground black pepper, as required
- 4 cups fresh mushrooms, chopped
- 1 tomato, chopped

- 3 ounces boneless cod fillet, chopped

- 1½ cups onion, sliced into rings

- 1 red bell pepper, seeded and chopped

- 1 green bell pepper, seeded and chopped

- 1/3 cup low-fat mozzarella, shredded

Instructions:

1. Preheat your oven to400 degrees F.

2. Grease a pie dish with cooking spray.

3. For base: in a large bowl, add all the ingredients and mix until well combined.

4. Transfer the mixture into prepared pie dish and press to smooth the surface.

5. Bake for about 40 minutes.

6. Remove from the oven and set aside to cool for at least 15 minutes.

7. Carefully turn out the crust onto a baking sheet.

8. For topping: in s bowl, add tomato paste, herbs and black pepper.

9. Spread tomato sauce mixture over crust evenly.

10. Arrange the vegetables over tomato sauce, followed by the cheese.

11. Transfer the baking sheet into the oven and bake for about 20 minutes or until cheese is melted.

12. Serve hot.

Chapter 6: Dinner Recipes

Chicken Taco Bowl

Yield: 4 servings

Preparation Time: 20 minutes

Cooking Time: 15 minutes

Total Time: 35 minutes

Ingredients:

For Chicken:

- 4 (4-ounce) boneless, skinless chicken breasts
- Freshly ground black pepper, as required
- 2 tablespoons olive oil
- ¾ cup low-fat chicken broth

For Topping:

- 1 cup cooked black beans
- 1 large avocado, peeled, pitted and sliced
- 1 large plum tomato, chopped
- 2 tablespoons jalapeno peppers, chopped
- ¼ cup low-fat Cheddar cheese, shredded
- 2 scallions, chopped
- 2 tablespoons fresh cilantro, chopped

Instructions:

1. Season the chicken breasts with salt and black pepper evenly.

2. Heat the oil in a large skillet over medium heat and cook the chicken breasts for about 5 minutes.

3. Flip the chicken breast and to with the broth.

4. Cook, covered for about 7-10 minutes or until cooked through.

5. With a slotted spoon, transfer the chicken breast into a bowl and with 2 forks, shred the meat.

6. Add any remaining liquid from the pan into the shredded chicken and stir to combine.

7. Divide the shredded chicken into serving bowls and serve with the topping ingredients.

Herbed Chicken Thighs

Yield: 6 servings

Preparation Time: 15 minutes

Cooking Time: 1 hour

Total Time: 1¼ hours

Ingredients:

- 6 bone-in chicken thighs
- Freshly ground black pepper, as required
- 2 tablespoons extra-virgin olive oil
- ½ of red onion, sliced
- 8 sprigs fresh rosemary
- ½ teaspoon cayenne pepper
- 4 cups low-fat chicken broth
- 2 tablespoons freshly squeezed lemon juice
- 2 tablespoons arrowroot starch
- 1 tablespoon cold filtered water
- ½ tablespoon fresh lemon zest, grated finely

Instructions:

1. Sprinkle the chicken thighs with black pepper evenly.
2. Heat the oil in a large skillet over high heat.
3. Place the chicken, skin side down and cook for about 3-4 minutes.
4. With a slotted spoon, transfer the chicken thighs onto a plate.

5. In the same skillet, add onion over medium heat and sauté for about 4-5 minutes.

6. Return the thighs in the skillet, skin side up.

7. Place the rosemary sprigs over thighs and sprinkle with cayenne pepper.

8. Add the broth and bring to a boil.

9. Decrease the heat to medium-low and simmer, covered for about 40-45 minutes, coating the thighs with cooking liquid occasionally.

10. Meanwhile, in a small bowl, dissolve the arrowroot starch in water.

11. Discard the rosemary sprigs and transfer the thighs into a bowl.

12. Add the lemon juice in sauce and stir to combine.

13. Slowly, add the arrowroot starch mixture in sauce, stirring continuously.

14. Cook for about 3-4 minutes or until desired thickness, stirring occasionally.

15. Pour the sauce over chicken thighs and serve hot with the topping of lemon zest.

Chicken with Bell Peppers

Yield: 6 servings

Preparation Time: 15 minutes

Cooking Time: 17 minutes

Total Time: 32 minutes

Ingredients:

- 6 (4-ounce) skinless, boneless chicken thighs
- Sea salt and freshly ground black pepper, as required
- 2 tablespoons extra-virgin olive oil, divided
- 1 white onion, chopped
- 1 red bell pepper, seeded and sliced thinly
- 1 orange bell pepper, seeded and sliced thinly
- 1 yellow bell pepper, seeded and sliced thinly
- 3 garlic cloves, minced
- 1 tablespoon fresh ginger, minced
- 1 teaspoon fresh orange peel, grated finely
- ½ cup freshly squeezed orange juice
- 1 cup raw cashews, toasted and chopped
- ½ cup scallions, sliced thinly

Instructions:

1. Season the chicken breasts with and salt and black pepper lightly.

2. In a large skillet, heat 1½ tablespoons of the oil over medium heat and cook the chicken breasts for about 2-3 minutes per side.

3. Add in the onion and bell peppers and cook for about 3-4 minutes.

4. With a slotted spoon, transfer the cooked chicken and bell pepper mixture into a larger bowl.

5. In the same skillet, heat the remaining oil over medium heat and sauté the garlic and ginger for about 1 minute.

6. Stir in the orange juice and cook for about 3 minutes or until juice reduces slightly.

7. Return the chicken and bell pepper mixture into the skillet.

8. Stir in the cashews and cook for about 2-3 minutes.

9. Serve hot with the garnishing of scallion.

Yogurt & Parmesan Chicken Bake

Yield: 4 servings

Preparation Time: 15 minutes

Cooking Time: 45 minutes

Total Time: 1 hour

Ingredients:

- 1 cup fat-free plain Greek yogurt
- ½ cup low-fat Parmesan cheese, grated
- 1 teaspoon garlic powder
- Freshly ground black pepper, as required
- 4 (4-ounce) boneless, skinless chicken breasts

Instructions:

1. Preheat your oven to375 degrees F.
2. Line baking sheet with a greased piece of foil.
3. In a bowl, add the yogurt, cheese, garlic powder and black pepper and mix well.
4. Add the chicken breasts and coat with the yogurt mixture evenly.
5. Arrange the chicken breasts onto the prepared baking sheet in a single layer.
6. Bake for about 45 minutes.
7. Serve hot.

Chicken & Broccoli Bake

Yield: 6 servings

Preparation Time: 15 minutes

Cooking Time: 24 minutes

Total Time: 39 minutes

Ingredients:

- Olive oil cooking spray
- 6 (6-ounce) skinless, boneless chicken thighs
- 3 broccoli heads, cut into florets
- 4 garlic cloves, minced
- ¼ cup extra-virgin olive oil
- 1 teaspoon dried oregano, crushed
- 1 teaspoon dried rosemary, crushed
- Sea salt and freshly ground black pepper, as required

Instructions:

1. Preheat your oven to375 degrees F. Grease a large baking dish with cooking spray.
2. In a large bowl, add all the ingredients and toss to coat well.
3. In the bottom of prepared baking dish, arrange the broccoli florets and top with chicken breasts in a single layer.
4. Bake for about 45 minutes.
5. Serve hot.

Chicken, Rice & Black Beans Casserole

Yield: 8 servings

Preparation Time: 20 minutes

Cooking Time: 1 hour 25 minutes

Total Time: 1 hour 45 minutes

Ingredients:

- 1/3 cup brown rice
- 1 cup low-fat vegetable broth
- Olive oil cooking spray
- 1 tablespoon olive oil
- 1/3 cup yellow onion, chopped
- 16 ounces cooked boneless, skinless chicken, cut into small pieces
- 1 medium zucchini, sliced thinly
- ½ cup fresh shiitake mushrooms, sliced
- ½ teaspoon ground cumin
- ¼ teaspoon cayenne pepper
- 1 (15-ounce) can black beans, drained and rinsed
- 1/3 cup carrots, peeled and shredded
- 1 (4-ounce) can diced green chilies
- 2 cups low-fat Swiss cheese, shredded

Instructions:

1. In a pan, add the rice and broth over medium-high heat and bring to a boil.
2. Decrease the heat to low and simmer, covered for about 45 minutes or until rice is tender.
3. Preheat oven to 350 degrees F. Lightly grease a large casserole dish with cooking spray.
4. Meanwhile, in a skillet, heat olive oil over medium heat and sauté the onion for about 4-5 minutes.
5. Stir in the chicken, zucchini, mushrooms, cumin and cayenne pepper and cook for about 4-5 minutes.
6. In a large bowl, add the cooked rice, chicken mixture, black beans, carrots, green chilies and 1 cup of Swiss cheese and mix well.
7. Transfer the chicken mixture into the prepared casserole dish evenly and sprinkle with the remaining Swiss cheese.
8. With a piece of foil, cover the casserole dish loosely and bake for about 30 minutes.
9. Uncover the casserole dish and bake for about 10 minutes or until top becomes lightly browned.
10. Remove from the oven and set aside for about 5 minutes before serving.

Chicken & Black Beans Chili

Yield: 6 servings

Preparation Time: 15 minutes

Cooking Time: 45 minutes

Total Time: 1 hour

Ingredients:

- 4 cups low-fat chicken broth, divided
- 3 cups cooked black beans, divided
- 1 tablespoon extra-virgin olive oil
- 1 large yellow onion, chopped
- 2 medium poblano peppers, seeded and chopped
- 1 jalapeño pepper, seeded and chopped
- 4 garlic cloves, minced
- 1 teaspoon dried thyme, crushed
- 1½ tablespoons ground coriander
- 1 tablespoon ground cumin
- ½ tablespoon ancho chili powder
- 4 cups cooked chicken, shredded
- 1 tablespoon freshly squeezed lime juice
- ¼ cup scallion (green part), chopped

Instructions:

1. In a food processor, add 1 cup of the broth and 1 can of black beans and pulse until smooth.
2. Transfer the beans puree into a bowl and set aside.

3. In a large pan, heat oil over medium heat and sauté the onion, poblano and jalapeño for about 4-5 minutes.

4. Add the garlic, thyme and spices and sauté for about 1 minute.

5. Stir in the bens puree and remaining broth and bring to a boil.

6. Decrease the heat to low and simmer for about 20 minutes.

7. Stir in the remaining can of beans, chicken and lime juice and bring to a boil.

8. Decrease the heat to low and simmer for about 5-10 minutes.

9. Serve hot with the topping of scallion greens.

Turkey Chili

Yield: 8 servings

Preparation Time: 15 minutes

Cooking Time: 2¼ hours

Total Time: 2½ hours

Ingredients:

- 2 tablespoons olive oil
- 1 small yellow onion, chopped
- 1 green bell pepper, seeded and chopped
- 4 garlic cloves, minced
- 1 jalapeño pepper, seeded and chopped
- 1 teaspoon dried thyme, crushed
- 2 tablespoons red chili powder
- 1 tablespoon ground cumin
- 2 pounds lean ground turkey
- 2 cups fresh tomatoes, chopped finely
- 2 ounces sugar-free tomato paste
- 2 cups low-fat chicken broth
- 1 cup water
- Freshly ground black pepper, as required
- ½ cup fresh cilantro, chopped

Instructions:

1. In a large Dutch oven, heat the oil over medium heat and sauté the onion and bell pepper for about 5-7 minutes.
2. Add the garlic, jalapeño pepper, thyme and spices and sauté for about 1 minute.
3. Add the turkey and cook for about 4-5 minutes.
4. Stir in the tomatoes, tomato paste and cacao powder and cook for about 2 minutes.
5. Add in the broth and water and bring to a boil.
6. Now, Decrease the heat to low and simmer, covered for about 2 hours.
7. Stir in the black pepper and remove from the heat.
8. Top with cilantro and serve hot.

Ground Turkey with Peas

Yield: 6 servings

Preparation Time: 15 minutes

Cooking Time: 40 minutes

Total Time: 55 minutes

Ingredients:

- 2 tablespoons extra virgin olive oil
- 1 pound lean ground turkey
- 1 large white onion, chopped finely
- 2 garlic cloves, minced
- ½ tablespoon fresh ginger, minced
- 1 teaspoon ground coriander
- 1 teaspoon ground cumin
- ¼ teaspoon chili powder
- 2 medium tomatoes, seeded and chopped
- ½ cup low-fat chicken broth
- Freshly ground black pepper, as required
- 2¼ cups fresh peas, shelled
- 2 tablespoons fresh cilantro, chopped

Instructions:

1. Heat the oil in a large skillet over medium heat and cook the turkey for about 4-5 minutes or until browned completely.

2. With a slotted spoon, transfer the turkey into a large bowl.

3. In the same skillet, add the onion and sauté for about 4-6 minutes.

4. Add the garlic, ginger, coriander, cumin and chili powder and sauté for about 1 minute.

5. Add the tomatoes and cook for about 2-3 minutes, crushing completely with the back of spoon.

6. Stir in the cooked turkey and broth and bring to a boil.

7. Decrease the heat to medium-low and simmer, covered for about 8-10 minutes, stirring occasionally.

8. Stir in peas and cook for about 15-20 minutes.

9. Remove from heat and serve hot with the garnishing of almonds and cilantro leaves.

Turkey & Spinach Pinwheel

Yield: 5 servings

Preparation Time: 20 minutes

Cooking Time: 1 hour

Total Time: 1 hour 20 minutes

Ingredients:

For Turkey Meatloaf:

- 1¼ pounds lean ground turkey
- 1 egg, beaten
- ¾ cup whole-wheat breadcrumbs
- Freshly ground black pepper, as required

For Filling:

- ¾ cup low-fat Parmesan cheese, shredded
- 1 (10-ounce) bag package frozen chopped spinach, thawed and drained
- 1 teaspoon Italian seasoning

For Topping:

- 3 tablespoons sugar-free tomato ketchup
- ¼ cup low-fat Parmesan cheese, shredded

Instructions:

1. Preheat your oven to350 degrees F. Arrange a rack into a roasting pan.
2. Line a baking sheet with a large parchment paper.
3. For meatloaf: in a large bowl, add all the ingredients and mix until well combined.
4. Place the turkey mixture onto the prepared baking sheet and with your hands, shape into a 10x14-inch sized rectangle.
5. With your hands, slightly, flatten the mixture.
6. For filling: in another bowl, add all the ingredients and gently, mix to combine.
7. Place the spinach mixture over turkey rectangle, leaving ¾-inch space from all sides.
8. Pick up the one edge of parchment paper and roll it over the meat, starting with the short end.
9. Continue to roll until the meat mixture form in a firm roll, by pulling back the parchment paper.
10. Place the roll, seam side down onto the rack in roasting pan.
11. Bake for about 50 minutes.
12. Remove the roasting pan from oven.
13. Place the ketchup over roll evenly and sprinkle with cheese evenly.
14. Bake for about 10 minutes more.
15. Remove from the oven and set aside to cool slightly before slicing.

16. With a sharp knife, cut the roll into desired sized slices
    and serve.

Veggies Stuffed Steak

Yield: 6 servings

Preparation Time: 15 minutes

Cooking Time: 35 minutes

Total Time: 50 minutes

Ingredients:

- Olive oil cooking spray
- 1 (1½-pound) flank steak, trimmed
- Salt and freshly ground black pepper, as required
- 1 tablespoon olive oil
- 2 small garlic cloves, minced
- 6 ounces fresh spinach, chopped finely
- 1 medium green bell pepper, seeded and chopped
- 1 medium tomato, chopped finely

Instructions:

1. Preheat your oven to425 degrees F. Grease a large baking dish with cooking spray.
2. Place the flank steak onto a clean cutting board.
3. Hold a sharp knife parallel to work surface, slice the steak horizontally, without cutting all the way through, that you can open like a book.
4. With a pounder, flatten the steak to an even thickness.
5. Sprinkle the steak with a little salt and black pepper evenly.

6. In a skillet, heat the oil over medium heat and sauté the garlic for about 1 minute.

7. Add spinach and cook for about 2 minutes.

8. Stir in the bell pepper and tomato and immediately remove from heat.

9. Transfer the spinach mixture into a bowl and set aside to cool slightly.

10. Place the filling on top of steak evenly.

11. Roll up the steak to seal the filling.

12. With cotton twine, tie the steak.

13. Place the steak roll into the prepared baking dish.

14. Roast for about 30-35 minutes.

15. Remove from the oven and let it cool slightly before slicing.

16. With a sharp knife, cut the roll into desired sized slices and serve.

Spicy Steak with Salsa

Yield: 4 servings

Preparation Time: 20 minutes

Cooking Time: 12 minutes

Total Time: 32 minutes

Ingredients:

For Steak:

- 2 garlic cloves, minced
- ½ teaspoon ground cumin
- ¼ teaspoon ground coriander
- ¼ teaspoon cayenne pepper
- Pinch of sea salt
- Freshly ground black pepper, as required
- 2 tablespoons freshly squeezed lemon juice
- 1 (1-pound) flank steak, trimmed
- Olive oil cooking spray

For Salsa:

- ¾ cup yellow grape tomatoes, quartered
- ¾ cup red grape tomatoes, quartered
- ¼ cup red onion, chopped
- 2 tablespoons fresh cilantro
- 1 tablespoon freshly squeezed lemon juice
- Pinch of sea salt

- Freshly ground black pepper, as required

Instructions:

1. For steak: in a large bowl, add all the garlic, spices, salt, black pepper and lemon juice and mix until well combined.
2. Add the steak and coat with the spice mixture generously.
3. Set aside at room temperature for about 25-30 minutes.
4. Preheat the grill to medium-high heat. Grease the grill grate with cooking spray.
5. Place the steak onto the grill and cook for about 6 minutes per side.
6. Remove the steak from grill and place onto a cutting board for about 10 minutes before slicing.
7. Meanwhile, for salsa: in a bowl, add all the ingredients and gently, stir to combine.
8. With a sharp knife, cut the steak into desired sized slices.
9. Divide the steak slices onto serving plates and serve with the topping of salsa.

Beef with Cauliflower

Yield: 4 servings

Preparation Time: 15 minutes

Cooking Time: 12 minutes

Total Time: 27 minutes

Ingredients:

- 1 tablespoon olive oil
- 4 garlic cloves, minced
- 1 pound beef sirloin steak, cut into bite sized pieces
- 3½ cups cauliflower florets
- 3 tablespoons low-fat chicken broth
- Freshly ground black pepper, as required
- ¼ cup fresh cilantro leaves, chopped

Instructions:

1. Heat the oil in a large skillet over medium heat and sauté the garlic for about 1 minute.
2. Add the beef pieces and stir to combine.
3. Increase the heat to medium-high and cook for about 6-8 minutes or until browned from all sides.
4. Meanwhile, in a pan of boiling water, add the cauliflower and cook for about 5-6 minutes.
5. Remove from the heat and drain the cauliflower completely.

6. Add the cauliflower and broth in skillet with beef and cook for about 2-3 minutes.

7. Stir in the black pepper and remove from the heat.

8. Serve hot with the garnishing of cilantro.

Baked Beef & Cauliflower Stew

Yield: 12 servings

Preparation Time: 15 minutes

Cooking Time: 2¼ hours

Total Time: 2½ hours

Ingredients:

- 1 teaspoon ground cumin
- 1 teaspoon ground coriander
- ½ teaspoon cayenne pepper
- ½ teaspoon ground cinnamon
- 3 pounds beef stew meat, trimmed and cubed
- Pinch of sea salt
- Freshly ground black pepper, as required
- 2 tablespoons extra-virgin olive oil
- 1 yellow onion, chopped
- 2 garlic cloves, minced
- 2¼ cups fat-free chicken broth
- 2 cups tomatoes, chopped finely
- 1 large head cauliflower, cut into small florets

Instructions:

1. Preheat your oven to300 degrees F.
2. In a small bowl, add all the spices and mix well. Set aside.
3. Season the beef with a pinch of salt and black pepper.

4. In a large ovenproof pan, heat the oil over medium heat and cook the beef cubes for about 10 minutes or until browned from all sides.

5. With a slotted spoon, transfer the beef cubes into a bowl.

6. In the same pan, add the onion and sauté for about 3-4 minutes.

7. Add the garlic and spice mixture and sauté for about 1 minute.

8. Add the cooked beef, broth and tomatoes and bring to a gentle boil.

9. Immediately, cover the pan and transfer into the oven.

10. Bake for about 1½ hours.

11. Remove the pan from oven and stir in the cauliflower.

12. Bake for about 30 minutes more or until cauliflower is done completely.

Beef & Carrot Curry

Yield: 4 servings

Preparation Time: 20 minutes

Cooking Time: 1 hour 50 minutes

Total Time: 2 hours 10 minutes

Ingredients:

- 2 teaspoons olive oil
- 1 pound boneless beef, trimmed and cubed into 1-inch size
- 1 celery stalk, chopped
- 1 medium onion, chopped
- 1/3 of red chili, chopped
- 2 garlic cloves, minced
- ½ teaspoon curry powder
- 2 teaspoons ground cumin
- ½ teaspoon ground turmeric
- 1 tablespoon tomato paste
- 1 cup fat-free plain Greek yogurt, whipped
- ½ cup water
- 1 large carrot, peeled and chopped
- 1 teaspoon fresh lime juice
- Freshly ground black pepper, as required
- 2 tablespoons fresh cilantro leaves, chopped

Instructions:

1. Heat the oil in a large pan over high heat and sear the beef cubes for about 4-5 minutes.
2. Add the onion, celery and red chili and cook for about 1 minute.
3. Decrease the heat to medium.
4. Stir in the garlic, curry powder and spices and cook for about 1 minute.
5. Stir in the tomato paste, yogurt and water and cook until boiling.
6. Decrease the heat to low and simmer, covered for about 1 hour, stirring occasionally.
7. Stir in the carrot and simmer, covered for about 40 minutes.
8. Stir in the lime juice and black pepper and remove from heat.
9. Serve hot with the garnishing f cilantro.

Baked Beef & Black Beans Chili

Yield: 4 servings

Preparation Time: 15 minutes

Cooking Time: 2 hours

Total Time: 2¼ hours

Ingredients:

- 1½ tablespoons extra-virgin olive oil, divided
- 1 cup white onion, chopped
- 6 large garlic cloves, minced
- 2 dried New Mexico chiles, stemmed, seeded and torn
- 3 dried ancho chiles, stemmed, seeded and torn
- 2 teaspoons dried oregano, crushed
- 1½ teaspoons ground cumin
- 2 large plum tomatoes, chopped
- 2 cups low-fat chicken broth
- 1 pound beef stew meat, trimmed and cubed
- Freshly ground black pepper, as required
- 1 (15-ounce) can black beans, rinsed and drained
- 2 tablespoons fresh cilantro, chopped

Instructions:

1. In an oven-proof pan, heat 1 tablespoon of the oil over medium heat and sauté the onion for about 4-5 minutes.
2. Add the garlic, both chiles, oregano and cumin and sauté for about 1 minute.

3. Add in the tomatoes and broth and bring to a boil.

4. Decrease the heat to medium-low and simmer, covered for about 30 minutes.

5. Preheat your oven to325 degrees F. Arrange a rack in the center of the oven.

6. Remove the pan from heat and set aside to cool slightly.

7. Transfer the chile mixture into a blender and pulse until pureed.

8. Return the chile puree into the same pan.

9. Meanwhile, in another pan, heat the remaining oil over medium-high heat and cook the beef black pepper for about 3-4 minutes.

10. Transfer the cooked beef into the pan with puree and stir to combine.

11. Cover the pan and immediately, transfer into the oven.

12. Bake for about 50 minutes.

13. Remove from the oven and place the pan over medium-low heat.

14. Stir in the beans and simmer, uncovered for about 30 minutes.

15. Serve hot with the garnishing of cilantro.

Ground Beef Chili

Yield: 8 servings

Preparation Time: 15 minutes

Cooking Time: 2¼ hours

Total Time: 2½ hours

Ingredients:

- 2 tablespoons extra-virgin olive oil
- 1 large white onion, chopped
- 1 large green bell pepper, seeded and chopped
- 4 garlic cloves, minced
- 1 jalapeño pepper, chopped
- 1 teaspoon dried thyme, crushed
- 1 teaspoon dried basil, crushed
- 2 tablespoons red chili powder
- 1 tablespoon ground cumin
- 1 teaspoon ground allspice
- 2 pounds lean ground beef
- 2 cups fresh tomatoes, chopped finely
- 1 (6-ounce) can sugar-free tomato paste
- 2 cups low-fat chicken broth
- 1 cup filtered water
- 4 scallions, chopped

Instructions:

1. Heat the oil in a large pan over medium heat and sauté the onion and bell pepper for about 5-7 minutes.
2. Add the garlic, jalapeño pepper, dried herbs, spices and black pepper and sauté for about 1 minute.
3. Add the beef and cook for about 4-5 minutes.
4. Stir in the tomatoes, tomato paste and cacao powder and cook for about 2 minutes.
5. Add the broth and water and cook until boiling.
6. Decrease the heat to low and simmer, covered for about 2 hours.
7. Serve hot with the garnishing of scallion.

Meatballs in Tomato Gravy

Yield: 5 servings

Preparation Time: 20 minutes

Cooking Time: 30 minutes

Total Time: 50 minutes

Ingredients:

For Meatballs:

- 1 pound lean ground beef
- 1 tablespoon tomato paste
- ¼ cup fresh cilantro leaves, chopped
- 1 small onion, chopped finely
- 2 garlic cloves, minced
- ½ teaspoon ground cumin
- Freshly ground black pepper, as required

For Tomato Gravy:

- 3 tablespoons extra-virgin olive oil, divided
- 2 medium red onions, chopped finely
- 2 garlic cloves, minced
- ½ tablespoon fresh ginger, minced
- 1 teaspoon dried thyme, crushed
- 1 teaspoon ground cumin
- 1 teaspoon cayenne pepper
- 3 large tomatoes, chopped finely

- Freshly ground black pepper, as required
- 1½ cups warm low-fat chicken broth
- 3 tablespoons fresh parsley, chopped

Instructions:

1. For meatballs: in a large bowl, add all the ingredients and mix until well combined.
2. Make small equal sized balls from the beef mixture and set aside.
3. For gravy: in a large pan, heat 1 tablespoon of the oil over medium heat and cook the meatballs for about 4-5 minutes or until lightly browned from all sides.
4. With a slotted spoon, transfer the meatballs onto a plate.
5. Heat the remaining oil in the same pan over medium heat and cook the onion for about 8-10 minutes, stirring frequently.
6. Add the garlic, ginger, thyme and spices and sauté for about 1 minute.
7. Add the tomatoes and cook for about 3-4 minutes, crushing with the back of spoon.
8. Add the warm broth and bring to a boil.
9. Carefully add meatballs and cook for about 5 minutes, without stirring.
10. Decrease the heat to low and simmer, partially covered for about 15-20 minutes, stirring carefully 2-3 times.
11. Serve hot with the garnishing of parsley.

Lemony Trout

Yield: 4 servings

Preparation Time: 15 minutes

Cooking Time: 25 minutes

Total Time: 40 minutes

Ingredients:

- 2 (1½-pound) wild-caught trout, gutted and cleaned
- Salt and freshly ground black pepper, as required
- 1 lemon, sliced
- 2 tablespoons fresh dill, minced
- 2 tablespoons olive oil
- 2 tablespoons freshly squeezed lemon juice

Instructions:

1. Preheat your oven to475 degrees F. Arrange a wire rack onto a foil-lined baking sheet.
2. Sprinkle the trout with salt and black pepper from inside and outside generously.
3. Fill the cavity of each fish with lemon slices and dill.
4. Place the trout onto the prepared baking sheet and drizzle with the melted butter and lemon juice.
5. Bake for about 25 minutes.
6. Remove the baking sheet from oven and transfer the trout onto a serving platter.

7. Serve hot.

Halibut with Veggies

Yield: 4 servings

Preparation Time: 15 minutes

Cooking Time: 20 minutes

Total Time: 35 minutes

Ingredients:

- Olive oil cooking spray
- 1 teaspoon olive oil
- ½ cup yellow onion, minced
- 1 cup zucchini, chopped
- 2 garlic cloves, minced
- 2 tablespoons fresh basil, chopped
- 2 cups fresh tomatoes, chopped
- Freshly ground black pepper, as required
- 4 (6-ounce) halibut steaks
- 1/3 cup feta cheese, crumbled

Instructions:

1. Preheat your oven to450 degrees F.
2. Grease a large shallow baking dish with cooking spray.
3. In a skillet, heat the oil over medium heat and sauté the onion, zucchini and garlic for about 4-5 minutes.
4. Stir in the basil, tomatoes and black pepper and immediately remove from heat.

5. Place the halibut steaks into prepared baking dish in a single layer.

6. Top with the tomato mixture evenly and sprinkle with cheese evenly.

7. Bake for about 15 minutes or until desired doneness.

8. Serve hot.

Cod with Olives & Tomatoes

Yield: 4 servings

Preparation Time: 15 minutes

Cooking Time: 15 minutes

Total Time: 30 minutes

Ingredients:

- 2 tablespoons extra-virgin olive oil
- 1 onion, sliced thinly
- 2 garlic cloves, minced
- ¾ cup low-fat chicken broth
- 1 tablespoon fresh parsley, chopped
- ½ cup black olives, pitted and sliced
- 2 cups tomatoes, chopped finely
- 1 pound cod fillets

Instructions:

1. Heat the oil in a large skillet over medium heat and sauté the onion and garlic for about 4-5 minutes.
2. Add the remaining ingredients except cod fillets and cook for about 5 minutes.
3. Stir in the cod fillets and cook for about 5 minutes or until desired doneness.
4. Serve hot.

Baked Salmon Parcel

Yield: 6 servings

Preparation Time: 15 minutes

Cooking Time: 20 minutes

Total Time: 35 minutes

Ingredients:

- 6 (3-ounce) fresh salmon fillets
- Sea salt and freshly ground black pepper, as required
- 1 yellow bell pepper, seeded and thinly sliced
- 1 red bell pepper, seeded and thinly sliced
- 1 green bell pepper, seeded and thinly sliced
- 12 cherry tomatoes, halved
- 1 small onion, sliced thinly
- ¼ cup fresh rosemary, chopped
- ¼ cup fresh dill, chopped
- ¼ cup extra-virgin olive oil
- 2 tablespoons freshly squeezed lemon juice

Instructions:

1. Preheat your oven to400 degrees F.
2. Arrange 6 pieces of foil onto a smooth surface.
3. Place 1 salmon fillet on each foil paper and sprinkle with sea salt and black pepper.
4. In a bowl, mix together bell peppers, tomatoes and onion.
5. Place veggie mixture over each fillet evenly.

6. Top with parsley and dill evenly.

7. Drizzle with oil and lemon juice.

8. Fold the foil around salmon mixture to seal it.

9. Arrange the foil packets onto a large baking sheet in a single layer.

10. Bake for about 20 minutes.

11. Remove from the oven and carefully, open the foil parcels.

12. Serve hot.

Salmon with Salsa

Yield: 2 servings

Preparation Time: 20 minutes

Cooking Time: 8 minutes

Total Time: 28 minutes

Ingredients:

For Salsa:

- 2 tablespoons red onion, chopped
- 1 cup fresh pineapple, chopped
- ½ cup red bell pepper, seeded and chopped
- 1 tablespoon freshly squeezed lemon juice
- Freshly ground black pepper, as required

For Salmon:

- 2 (5-ounce) (1-inch thick) salmon fillets
- Sea salt and freshly ground black pepper, as required
- 1 tablespoon extra-virgin olive oil
- 2 tablespoons fresh cilantro leaves, chopped

Instructions:

1. For salsa: in a bowl, add all the ingredients and gently, stir to combine.
2. Cover the bowl and refrigerate until serving.
3. Season the salmon fillets with salt and black pepper evenly.

4. Heat the oil in a large skillet over medium-high heat.

5. Place the salmon, skins side up and cook for about 4 minutes.

6. Carefully, change the side of fillets and cook for about 4 minutes more.

7. Divide the salmon fillets onto serving plates and serve with the topping of salsa.

Herbed Salmon & Shrimp Stew

Yield: 8 servings

Preparation Time: 20 minutes

Cooking Time: 21 minutes

Total Time: 41 minutes

Ingredients:

- 2 tablespoons olive oil
- ½ cup white onion, chopped finely
- 2 garlic cloves, minced
- 1 Serrano pepper, seeded and chopped
- 1 teaspoon smoked paprika
- 4 cups fresh tomatoes, chopped
- 4 cups low-fat chicken broth
- 1½ pounds salmon fillets, cubed
- 1 pound shrimp, peeled and deveined
- 2 tablespoons freshly squeezed lime juice
- ¼ cup fresh basil, chopped
- ¼ cup fresh parsley, chopped
- Freshly ground black pepper, as required
- 2 scallions, chopped

Instructions:

1. Heat the oil in a large soup pan over medium-high heat and sauté the onion for about 5-6 minutes.

2. Add the garlic, Serrano pepper and smoked paprika and sauté for about 1 minute.

3. Add in the tomatoes and broth and bring to a gentle simmer over medium heat.

4. Simmer for about 5 minutes.

5. Add the salmon and simmer for about 3-4 minutes.

6. Stir in the shrimp and cook for about 4-5 minutes.

7. Stir in the lemon juice, basil, parsley and black pepper and remove from heat.

8. Serve hot with the garnishing of scallion.

Shrimp & Tomato Casserole

Yield: 6 servings

Preparation Time: 20 minutes

Cooking Time: 25 minutes

Total Time: 45 minutes

Ingredients:

- 2 tablespoon extra-virgin olive oil
- 1 tablespoon garlic, minced
- 1½ pounds large shrimp, peeled and deveined
- ¾ teaspoon dried oregano, crushed
- ½ teaspoon red pepper flakes, crushed
- ¼ cup fresh parsley, chopped
- ¾ cup low-fat chicken broth
- 1 tablespoon freshly squeezed lemon juice
- 2 cups tomatoes, chopped
- 4 ounces feta cheese, crumbled

Instructions:

1. Preheat your oven to350 degrees F.
2. Heat the oil in a large skillet over medium-high heat and sauté the garlic for about 1 minute.
3. Add the shrimp, oregano and red pepper flakes and cook for about 4-5 minutes.
4. Stir in the parsley and salt and immediately remove from the heat.

5. Transfer the shrimp mixture into a casserole dish and spread in an even layer.

6. In the same skillet, add the broth and lemon juice over medium heat and simmer for about 3-5 minutes or until reduces to half.

7. Stir in the tomatoes and cook for about 2-3 minutes.

8. Remove from the heat and place the tomato mixture over shrimp mixture evenly.

9. Top with feta cheese evenly.

10. Bake for about 15-20 minutes or until top becomes golden brown.

11. Serve hot.

Scallops with Broccoli

Yield: 5 servings

Preparation Time: 15 minutes

Cooking Time: 10 minutes

Total Time: 25 minutes

Ingredients:

For Broccoli:

- 1¼ pounds small broccoli florets

For Scallops:

- 1 tablespoon olive oil
- 2 garlic cloves, minced
- 1 pound fresh jumbo scallops, side muscles removed
- Salt and freshly ground black pepper, as required
- 2 tablespoons freshly squeezed lemon juice
- 2 scallions (green part), sliced thinly

Instructions:

1. For broccoli: arrange a steamer basket in a pan of water over medium-high heat and bring to a boil.
2. Place the broccoli in steamer basket and steam, covered for about 4-5 minutes.

3. Meanwhile, for scallops: Heat the oil in a large non-stick skillet over medium-high heat and sauté the garlic for about 1 minute.

4. Now, add the scallops and cook for about 2 minutes per side.

5. Stir in the salt, black pepper, and lemon juice and remove from heat.

6. Drain the broccoli and transfer onto serving plates.

7. Top with the scallops and serve immediately with the garnishing of scallions.

Scallops with Asparagus

Yield: 4 servings

Preparation Time: 15 minutes

Cooking Time: 10 minutes

Total Time: 25 minutes

Ingredients:

- 2 tablespoons olive oil
- ¼ cup shallot, chopped
- 2 garlic cloves, minced
- 2 tablespoons fresh rosemary, chopped finely
- 1 pound fresh asparagus, trimmed and cut into 1-inch pieces
- 2 teaspoons fresh lemon zest, grated finely
- 1½ pounds baby scallops, side muscles removed
- Sea salt and freshly ground black pepper, as required
- 2 tablespoons freshly squeezed lemon juice

Instructions:

1. Heat the oil in a large skillet over medium-high heat and sauté the shallot for about 2 minutes.
2. Add the garlic and rosemary and sauté for about 1 minute.
3. Add the asparagus and lemon zest and cook for about 1-2 minutes.

4. Stir in the scallops and immediately, Decrease the heat to medium.

5. Cover the skillet and cook for about 4-5 minutes, stirring occasionally.

6. Stir in the lemon juice, salt and black pepper and remove from the heat.

7. Serve hot.

Lentils & Quinoa Stew

Yield: 6 servings

Preparation Time: 15 minutes

Cooking Time: 33 minutes

Total Time: 48 minutes

Ingredients:

- 1 tablespoon extra-virgin olive oil
- 3 carrots, peeled and chopped
- 3 celery stalks, chopped
- 1 yellow onion, chopped
- 4 garlic cloves, minced
- 4 cups fresh tomatoes, chopped
- 1 cup red lentils, rinsed and drained
- ½ cup dried quinoa, rinsed and drained
- 1½ teaspoons ground cumin
- 1 teaspoon red chili powder
- 5 cups low-fat vegetable broth
- 2 cups fresh spinach, chopped

Instructions:

1. Heat the oil in a large pan over medium heat and cook the celery, onion and carrot for about 8 minutes, stirring frequently.
2. Add in the garlic and sauté for about 1 minute.

3. Add the remaining ingredients except spinach and bring to a boil.
4. Decrease the heat to low and simmer, covered for about 20 minutes.
5. Stir in spinach and simmer for about 3-4 minutes.
6. Serve hot.

Lentil Chili

Yield: 8 servings

Preparation Time: 15 minutes

Cooking Time: 2 hours 10 minutes

Total Time: 2 hours 25 minutes

Ingredients:

- 2 teaspoons extra-virgin olive oil
- 1 large white onion, chopped
- 2 medium carrots, peeled and chopped
- 2 celery stalks, chopped
- 1 large bell pepper, seeded and chopped
- 2 garlic cloves, minced
- 1 jalapeño pepper, seeded and chopped
- 1 tablespoon chipotle chili powder
- 1½ tablespoons ground coriander
- 1½ tablespoons ground cumin
- Freshly ground black pepper, as required
- 1 pound red lentils, rinsed
- 2 tablespoons tomato paste
- 8 cups low-fat vegetable broth
- 4 cups fresh spinach, torn
- ¼ cup fresh mint leaves, chopped
- ¼ cup fresh cilantro, chopped

Instructions:

1. Heat the oil in a large pan over medium heat and sauté the onion, carrot and celery for about 5 minutes.
2. Add the garlic, jalapeño pepper and spices and sauté for about 1 minute.
3. Add tomato paste, lentils and broth and bring to a boil.
4. Decrease the heat to low and simmer for about 2 hours.
5. Stir in the spinach and simmer for about 3-4 minutes.
6. Serve hot with the garnishing of mint and cilantro.

Quinoa with Green Beans

Yield: 4 servings

Preparation Time: 15 minutes

Cooking Time: 25 minutes

Total Time: 40 minutes

Ingredients:

- 3 tablespoons olive oil, divided
- 1 small onion, chopped
- 2 garlic cloves, minced
- 1 cup dried quinoa, rinsed
- Freshly ground black pepper, as required
- 1¾ cups low-fat vegetable broth
- 1 pound fresh green beans, trimmed and cut into 2-inch pieces
- 2 tablespoons freshly squeezed lemon juice
- 2 tablespoons fresh cilantro, chopped

Instructions:

1. Heat 1 tablespoon of the oil in a pan over medium heat and sauté the onion for about 2-3 minutes.
2. Add the garlic and sauté for about 1 minute.
3. Add the quinoa and cook for about 1 minute, stirring continuously.
4. Stir in the black pepper and broth and bring to a boil.

5. Decrease the heat to low and simmer, covered for about 15 minutes.
6. Remove from heat and set the pan aside, covered for about 10 minutes.
7. With a fork, fluff the quinoa.
8. Meanwhile, in a pan of the boiling water, add beans and cook for about 4-5 minutes.
9. Remove from the heat and drain the green beans well.
10. In a large serving bowl, add the quinoa, green beans, lemon juice, remaining oil and black pepper and toss to coat well.
11. Garnish with cilantro and serve.

Chapter 7: Snacks Recipes

Roasted Almonds

Yield: 4 servings

Preparation Time: 10 minutes

Cooking Time: 20 minutes

Total Time: 30 minutes

Ingredients:

- 1 cup whole almonds
- ¼ teaspoon ground cinnamon
- Freshly ground black pepper, as required
- ½ tablespoon extra-virgin olive oil

Instructions:

1. Preheat your oven to350 degrees F.
2. Line a baking sheet with a parchment paper.
3. In a bowl, add all ingredients and toss to coat well.
4. Transfer the almond mixture into prepared baking dish and spread in a single layer.
5. Roast for about 10 minutes, flipping twice.
6. Remove the baking sheet from oven and set aside to cool completely before serving.
7. You can preserve these roasted almonds in an airtight container at room temperature.

Roasted Walnuts

Yield: 8 servings

Preparation Time: 10 minutes

Cooking Time: 12 minutes

Total Time: 22 minutes

Ingredients:

- 2 cups walnuts pieces
- 2 tablespoons olive oil

Instructions:

1. Preheat your oven to375 degrees F.
2. Line a baking sheet with parchment paper.
3. In a bowl, add the walnuts and oil and toss to coat well.
4. Transfer the walnuts onto the prepared baking sheet and spread in a single layer.
5. Bake for about 12 minutes, stirring once halfway through.
6. Remove the baking sheet from oven and set aside to cool completely before serving.
7. You can store these walnuts in an airtight container at room temperature.

Cottage Cheese & Tomato Bowl

Yield: 2 servings

Preparation Time: 15 minutes

Total Time: 15 minutes

Ingredients:

- ¼ cup low-fat cottage cheese
- 1 tablespoon fresh basil, minced
- Pinch of freshly ground black pepper
- 10 cherry tomatoes, chopped

Instructions:

1. Add all ingredients in a bowl and stir to combine.
2. Serve immediately.

Carrot Sticks with Pesto

Yield: 14 servings

Preparation Time: 15 minutes

Cooking Time: 25 minutes

Total Time: 40 minutes

Ingredients:

For Carrot Sticks:

- Olive oil cooking spray
- 12 large carrots, peeled and cut into 2-inch long sticks

For Pesto:

- 2 garlic cloves, chopped
- ½ of jalapeño pepper, chopped roughly
- 1 cup fresh basil, chopped
- 1 tablespoon freshly squeezed lime juice
- 1 teaspoon ground cumin
- Pinch of sea salt
- Freshly ground black pepper, as required
- ¼ cup olive oil

Instructions:

1. Preheat your oven to 400 degrees F.
2. Lightly, grease 2 large baking sheets with cooking spray.

3. Divide the carrot sticks onto the prepared baking sheets evenly and arrange in a single layer.

4. Spray the carrot sticks with the cooking spray evenly.

5. Roast for about 20 minutes.

6. In the meantime, for pesto: in a food processor, add all the ingredients except oil and pulse until smooth.

7. While motor is running, slowly, add the oil and pulse until smooth.

8. Remove the carrot sticks from oven and toss with pesto.

9. Roast for 5 minutes more.

10. Remove from the oven and set aside to cool slightly.

11. Serve warm.

Cauliflower Poppers

Yield: 4 servings

Preparation Time: 15 minutes

Cooking Time: 30 minutes

Total Time: 45 minutes

Ingredients:

- Olive oil cooking spray
- 4 cups cauliflower florets
- 2 teaspoons olive oil
- ¼ teaspoon red chili powder
- Salt and freshly ground black pepper, as required

Instructions:

1. Preheat your oven to450 degrees F.
2. Grease a roasting pan with cooking spray.
3. In a bowl, add all ingredients and toss to coat well.
4. Transfer the cauliflower mixture into prepared roasting pan and spread in an even layer.
5. Roast for about 25-30 minutes.
6. Serve warm.

Sweet Potato Fries

Yield: 2 servings

Preparation Time: 10 minutes

Cooking Time: 25 minutes

Total Time: 35 minutes

Ingredients:

- 1 large sweet potato, peeled and cut into wedges
- 1 teaspoon ground turmeric
- 1 teaspoon ground cinnamon
- Pinch of sea salt
- Freshly ground black pepper, as required
- 2 tablespoons extra-virgin olive oil

Instructions:

1. Preheat your oven to 425 degrees F.
2. Line a baking sheet with a foil paper.
3. In a large bowl, add all the ingredients and toss to coat well.
4. Transfer the mixture into prepared baking sheet.
5. Bake for about 25 minutes, flipping once after 15 minutes.
6. Serve immediately.

Sweet Potato Croquettes

Yield: 4 servings

Preparation Time: 15 minutes

Cooking Time: 30 minutes

Total Time: 45 minutes

Ingredients:

- 3 cups cooked sweet potato, peeled and chopped roughly
- 2 tablespoons almond butter
- Pinch of sea salt
- 2 organic eggs
- 1 cup almond meal

Instructions:

1. Preheat your oven to 400 degrees F.
2. Line a large baking sheet with parchment paper.
3. In a bowl, add the sweet potato and with a fork mash it.
4. Add the almond butter and salt and mix well.
5. In a shallow, dish crack the eggs and beat well.
6. In another shallow dish, place the almond meal.
7. With a tablespoon of the sweet potato mixture, make balls and flatten each slightly.
8. Dip the croquettes in beaten eggs and then roll in almond meal completely.

9. Arrange the croquettes onto the prepared baking sheet in
    a single layer.

10. Bake for about 25-30 minutes or until done completely.

11. Serve warm.

Yogurt Deviled Eggs

Yield: 6 servings

Preparation Time: 15 minutes

Cooking Time: 20 minutes

Total Time: 35 minutes

Ingredients:

- 6 large eggs
- ¼ cup fat-free plain Greek yogurt
- 2 tablespoons scallions, chopped finely
- 1 tablespoon fresh chives, minced
- 1 tablespoon Dijon mustard
- Cayenne pepper, as required

Instructions:

1. In a pan of the water, add eggs and cook for about 15-20 minutes.
2. Remove from the heat and drain the eggs.
3. Set aside to cool completely.
4. Peel the eggs and with a sharp knife, slice them in half vertically.
5. Carefully, scoop out the yolks from each egg half.
6. In a blender, add the egg yolks and yogurt and pulse until smooth.
7. Transfer the yogurt mixture into a bowl.
8. Add the scallion, chives and mustard and stir to combine.

9. Spoon the yogurt mixture in each egg half evenly.

10. Serve with the sprinkling of cayenne pepper.

Green Deviled Eggs

Yield: 4 servings

Preparation Time: 15 minutes

Cooking Time: 20 minutes

Total Time: 35 minutes

Ingredients:

- 4 large eggs
- 1 medium avocado, peeled, pitted and chopped
- 2 teaspoons freshly squeezed lime juice
- Pinch of sea salt
- Cayenne pepper, as required

Instructions:

1. In a pan of the water, add the eggs and cook for about 15-20 minutes.
2. Remove from the heat and drain the eggs.
3. Set aside to cool completely.
4. Peel the eggs and with a sharp knife, slice them in half vertically.
5. Carefully, scoop out the yolks from each egg half.
6. In a bowl, add half of the egg yolks, avocado, lime juice and salt and with a fork, mash until well combined.
7. Spoon the avocado mixture in each egg half evenly.
8. Serve with the sprinkling of cayenne pepper.

Garlicky Chicken Wings

Yield: 8 servings

Preparation Time: 15 minutes

Cooking Time: 31 minutes

Total Time: 46 minutes

Ingredients:

- 3 pounds chicken wings
- 1½ tablespoons baking powder
- Salt and freshly ground black pepper, as required
- 2 tablespoons olive oil
- 4 garlic cloves, minced
- 2 teaspoons dried parsley flakes
- ½ teaspoon red pepper flakes, crushed
- 2 tablespoons fresh parsley, chopped

Instructions:

1. Preheat your oven to250 degrees F. Arrange a rack in lower third of oven. Place a greased rack onto foil-lined baking sheet.
2. In a bowl, add the wings, baking powder, salt and black pepper and toss to coat well.
3. Arrange the wings over prepared rack into baking sheet in a single layer.
4. Bake for about 30 minutes.

5. Remove the chicken wings from oven and transfer into a large bowl.

6. In a small frying pan, heat the oil over medium heat and sauté the garlic, dried parsley and red pepper flakes for about 20-30 seconds.

7. Remove from the heat and immediately, pour over chicken wings.

8. Add in the parsley and toss to coat well.

9. Serve immediately.

Buffalo Chicken Wings

Yield: 6 servings

Preparation Time: 15 minutes

Cooking Time: 20 minutes

Total Time: 35 minutes

Ingredients:

- 2 pounds chicken wings
- ¼ cup red hot sauce
- 2 tablespoons extra-virgin olive oil
- 1 teaspoon cayenne pepper
- Freshly ground black pepper, as required

Instructions:

1. Carefully, cut off the wing tips and then, cut each wing at the joint.
2. In a large bowl, add the hot sauce, oil, cayenne pepper and black pepper and mix until well combined.
3. In a cup, add 2 tablespoons of marinade and reserve it.
4. In the bowl of remaining marinade, add chicken wings and toss to coat well.
5. Set aside at room temperature for about 30 minutes.
6. Preheat your oven to broiler. Arrange a rack about 4-5-inch from the heating element.
7. Remove the wings from bowl and discard the marinade.

8. Arrange the wings over the rack of a broiler pan.

9. Broil for about 10 minutes per side.

10. Remove chicken wings from oven and coat with reserved marinade.

11. Serve immediately.

Chicken Nuggets

Yield: 4 servings

Preparation Time: 15 minutes

Cooking Time: 10 minutes

Total Time: 25 minutes

Ingredients:

- 2 large eggs
- 1½ cups blanched almond flour
- ½ cup tapioca flour
- ½ teaspoon paprika
- Pinch of sea salt
- Freshly ground black pepper, as required
- 2 skinless, boneless chicken breasts, cut into nuggets shape
- 3-4 tablespoons olive oil

Instructions:

1. In a shallow dish, crack the eggs and beat well.
2. In another shallow dish, add the flours, paprika, salt and black pepper and mix well.
3. Dip the chicken nuggets in beaten eggs and then coat with the flour mixture completely.

4. Heat the oil in a large non-stick skillet over medium-high heat and cook the chicken nuggets for about 4-5 minutes per side or until golden brown.

5. With a slotted spoon, transfer the nuggets onto a paper towel-lined plate to drain.

6. Serve warm.

Blueberry Bites

Yield: 10 servings

Preparation Time: 15 minutes

Total Time: 15 minutes

Ingredients:

- 1 scoop unsweetened protein powder
- ½ cup coconut flour, sifted
- 1-2 tablespoons powdered Erythritol
- ¼ teaspoon ground cinnamon
- ¼ cup dried blueberries
- ½-1 cup unsweetened almond milk

Instructions:

1. Line a large baking sheet with parchment paper. Set aside.
2. In a large bowl, add all the ingredients except almond milk and mix well.
3. Gradually, add desired amount of almond milk and mix until a dough is formed.
4. Immediately, make desired sized balls from mixture.
5. Arrange the balls onto the prepared baking sheet in a single layer.
6. Refrigerate to set for about 30 minutes before serving.

Almond Scones

Yield: 6 servings

Preparation Time: 10 minutes

Cooking Time: 20 minutes

Total Time: 30 minutes

Ingredients:

- Olive oil cooking spray
- 1 cup almonds
- 1 1/3 cups almond flour
- ¼ cup arrowroot flour
- 1 tablespoon coconut flour
- 1 teaspoon ground turmeric
- Pinch of sea salt
- Freshly ground black pepper, as required
- 1 egg
- ¼ cup olive oil
- 3 tablespoons raw honey
- 1 teaspoon vanilla extract

Instructions:

1. Preheat your oven to350 degrees F.
2. Lightly, grease a baking sheet with cooking spray.
3. In a food processor, add the almonds and pulse until chopped roughly

4. Transfer the chopped almonds into a large bowl.

5. Add the flours, turmeric, salt and black pepper and mix well.

6. In another bowl, place the remaining ingredients and beat until well combined.

7. Add the flour mixture into egg mixture and mix until well combined.

8. Arrange a plastic wrap over a cutting board.

9. Place the dough over cutting board.

10. With your hands, pat the dough into about 1-inch thick circle.

11. Carefully, cut the circle in 6 wedges.

12. Arrange the scones onto the prepared baking sheet in a single layer.

13. Bake for about 15-20 minutes.

14. Serve warm.

Quinoa Crackers

Yield: 6 servings

Preparation Time: 15 minutes

Cooking Time: 20 minutes

Total Time: 35 minutes

Ingredients:

- 3 tablespoons filtered water
- 1 tablespoon chia seeds
- 3 tablespoons sunflower seeds
- 1 tablespoon quinoa flour
- 1 teaspoon ground turmeric
- Pinch of ground cinnamon
- Pinch of sea salt

Instructions:

1. Preheat your oven to345 degrees F. Line a baking sheet with parchment paper.
2. In a bowl, add the water and chia seeds and soak for about 15 minutes.
3. After 15 minutes, add remaining ingredients and mix well.
4. Spread the mixture onto the prepared baking sheet and with the back of a spoon, smooth the top surface.
5. With a knife, cut the dough into small sized crackers.

6. Bake for about 20 minutes.

7. Remove the baking sheet from oven and set aside to cool completely before serving.

Lentil, Oats & Veggie Bites

Yield: 8 servings

Preparation Time: 15 minutes

Cooking Time: 1 hour

Total Time: 1¼ hours

Ingredients:

- 2¼ cups filtered water
- ½ cup green lentils
- 2 teaspoons olive oil
- 2 garlic cloves, minced
- 2 cups cremini mushrooms, chopped finely
- 1 cup fresh spinach, chopped finely
- ½ teaspoon fresh thyme, minced
- ½ teaspoon fresh rosemary, minced
- 1/3 cup dried unsweetened cranberries, chopped finely
- ½ cup walnut, toasted and chopped finely
- 1 tablespoon freshly squeezed lemon juice
- 1 egg, beaten
- ½ cup rolled oats, roughly ground
- Pinch of sea salt
- Pinch of red pepper flakes, crushed

Instructions:

1. In a large pan, add water and lentil over high heat and bring to a boil.
2. Decrease the heat to medium and simmer for about 20 minutes.
3. Remove from the heat and transfer the lentils into a bowl.
4. With a potato masher, mash the lentils until a coarse paste forms. Keep aside.
5. Preheat your oven to 350 degrees F.
6. Line a large baking sheet with a parchment paper
7. In the meantime, heat the oil in a large skillet over medium-high heat and sauté the garlic for about 1 minute.
8. Add the mushrooms and cook for about 8-9 minutes.
9. Add the spinach, herbs, cranberries, walnuts and lemon juice and cook for about 2 minutes.
10. Stir in the mashed lentils and immediately remove from heat.
11. Set aside to cool slightly.
12. Add the ground oats, salt and red pepper flakes and mix until well combined.
13. Make desired sized balls from the mixture.
14. Arrange the balls onto the prepared baking sheet in a single layer.
15. Bake for about 15 minutes.
16. Gently, change the side of balls and bake for about 13 minutes more.

17. Serve warm.

Berries Gazpacho

Yield: 6 servings

Preparation Time: 10 minutes

Total Time: 10 minutes

Ingredients:

- 2 cups fresh strawberries, hulled and sliced
- 2 cups fresh raspberries
- 4 cups unsweetened almond milk
- ½ teaspoon vanilla extract

Instructions:

- Add all ingredients in a food processor and pulse until smooth.
- Serve immediately.

Avocado Gazpacho

Yield: 6 servings

Preparation Time: 15 minutes

Total Time: 15 minutes

Ingredients:

- 3 large avocados, peeled, pitted and chopped
- 1/3 cup fresh cilantro leaves
- 3 cups fat-free vegetable broth
- 2 tablespoons freshly squeezed lemon juice
- 1 teaspoon ground cumin
- ¼ teaspoon cayenne pepper

Instructions:

1. Add all ingredients in a high-speed blender and pulse until smooth.
2. Transfer the soup into a large bowl.
3. Cover the bowl and refrigerate to chill for at least 2-3 hours before serving.

Black Beans Hummus

Yield: 10 servings

Preparation Time: 10 minutes

Total Time: 10 minutes

Ingredients:

- 15 ounces canned black beans, drained and rinsed
- ¼ cup salsa
- 2 garlic cloves, chopped
- 3 tablespoons tahini
- 2 cups boiled cauliflower
- 1 teaspoon ground cumin
- 1 teaspoon hot sauce
- 1 teaspoon extra-virgin olive oil

Instructions:

1. Add all ingredients in a blender and pulse until smooth.
2. Transfer into a bowl and serve.

Eggplant Caviar

Yield: 4 servings

Preparation Time: 15 minutes

Cooking Time: 20 minutes

Total Time: 35 minutes

Ingredients:

- Olive oil cooking spray
- 2½ pounds eggplants, halved lengthwise
- 2 garlic cloves, chopped
- ½ cup scallion, chopped
- 2 teaspoons fresh basil leaves
- 2 tablespoons salt-free vegetable broth
- 1 tablespoon freshly squeezed lemon juice
- Pinch of freshly ground black pepper
- 2½ teaspoons extra-virgin olive oil

Instructions:

1. Preheat your oven to400 degrees F.
2. Grease a baking sheet with cooking spray.
3. Place eggplant halves onto the prepared baking sheet, cut-side facing down.
4. Roast for about 20 minutes.
5. Remove the baking sheet from oven and let them cool slightly.

6. With a spoon, scoop out the pulp from skin.

7. In a food processor, add eggplant pulp and remaining ingredients except for oil and pulse until smooth.

8. Transfer the caviar into a bowl.

9. Add the olive oil and stir to combine.

10. Serve at room temperature.

Chapter 8: Smoothies & Juices Recipes

Protein Smoothie

Yield: 2 servings

Preparation Time: 10 minutes

Total Time: 10 minutes

Ingredients:

- ½ cup unsweetened vanilla whey protein powder
- 4 tablespoons almond butter
- 2 teaspoons vanilla extract
- 6-8 drops liquid stevia
- 2 cups unsweetened almond milk
- ¼ cup ice cubes

Instructions:

1. Add all ingredients in a high-speed blender and pulse until smooth.
2. Pour the smoothie into 2 serving glasses and serve immediately.

Tofu & Blueberries Smoothie

Yield: 2 servings

Preparation Time: 10 minutes

Total Time: 10 minutes

Ingredients:

- 8 ounces silken tofu, pressed and drained
- 1 large banana, peeled and sliced
- 1¼ cups unsweetened soy milk
- 1¼ cups frozen blueberries, divided
- 1 tablespoon honey
- ¼ cup ice cubes

Instructions:

1. Add all ingredients in a high-speed blender and pulse until smooth.
2. Pour the smoothie into 2 serving glasses and serve immediately.

Tofu & Mango Smoothie

Yield: 2 servings

Preparation Time: 10 minutes

Total Time: 10 minutes

Ingredients:

- 6 ounces silken tofu, pressed and drained
- 1½ cups frozen mango, peeled, pitted and chopped
- 1 large frozen banana, peeled
- ½ teaspoon ground turmeric
- ½ cup freshly squeezed orange juice
- 1 cup unsweetened almond milk

Instructions:

1. Add all ingredients in a high-speed blender and pulse until smooth.
2. Pour the smoothie into 2 serving glasses and serve immediately.

Oats & Mango Smoothie

Yield: 2 servings

Preparation Time: 10 minutes

Total Time: 10 minutes

Ingredients:

- ½ cup old-fashioned rolled oats
- 1 cup fat-free plain Greek yogurt
- 2 bananas, peeled and sliced
- 1 cup unsweetened almond milk
- ¼ teaspoon ground cinnamon

Instructions:

1. Add all ingredients in a high-speed blender and pulse until smooth.
2. Pour the smoothie into 2 serving glasses and serve immediately.

Oats & Mango Smoothie

Yield: 2 servings

Preparation Time: 10 minutes

Total Time: 10 minutes

Ingredients:

- 2 cups mango, peeled, pitted and chopped
- ¼ cup quick oats
- ¾ cup low-fat cottage cheese
- 1 tablespoon raw honey
- 1½ cups unsweetened almond milk
- ¼ cup ice cubes

Instructions:

1. Add all ingredients in a high-speed blender and pulse until smooth.
2. Pour the smoothie into 2 serving glasses and serve immediately.

Banana & Spinach Smoothie

Yield: 4 servings

Preparation Time: 10 minutes

Total Time: 10 minutes

Ingredients:

- 4 cups fresh spinach
- 4 large bananas, peeled and sliced
- 5 cups unsweetened almond milk
- ½ cup ice cubes

Instructions:

1. Add all ingredients in a high-speed blender and pulse until smooth.
2. Pour the smoothie into 4 serving glasses and serve immediately.

Mixed Fruit Smoothie

Yield: 3 servings

Preparation Time: 10 minutes

Total Time: 10 minutes

Ingredients:

- 1 avocado, peeled, pitted and chopped
- 1 cup frozen peach, pitted and chopped
- 1½ cups frozen strawberries, hulled
- 1½ cups frozen blackberries
- 2½ cups fat-free plain Greek yogurt
- ½ cup unsweetened almond milk

Instructions:

1. Add all ingredients in a high-speed blender and pulse until smooth.
2. Pour the smoothie into 3 serving glasses and serve immediately.

Blueberry & Lettuce Smoothie

Yield: 2 servings

Preparation Time: 10 minutes

Total Time: 10 minutes

Ingredients:

- 1 cup fresh blueberries
- 1½ cups romaine lettuce, chopped
- 4-6 drops liquid stevia
- 1½ cups unsweetened almond milk
- ½ cup ice cubes

Instructions:

1. Add all ingredients in a high-speed blender and pulse until smooth.
2. Pour the smoothie into 2 serving glasses and serve immediately.

Pumpkin Protein Smoothie

Yield: 2 servings

Preparation Time: 10 minutes

Total Time: 10 minutes

Ingredients:

- ¼ cup homemade pumpkin puree
- 1 frozen banana, peeled and sliced
- 1 scoop unsweetened vanilla protein powder
- ½ teaspoon vanilla extract
- ¼ teaspoon ground cinnamon
- 1¼ cups unsweetened soy milk
- ¼ cup ice cubes

Instructions:

1. Add all ingredients in a high-speed blender and pulse until smooth.
2. Pour the smoothie into 2 serving glasses and serve immediately.

Green Veggies Smoothie

Yield: 2 servings

Preparation Time: 10 minutes

Total Time: 10 minutes

Ingredients:

- 2 cups romaine lettuce, chopped
- 1 cup fresh baby spinach
- 1 cup fresh baby kale, tough ribs removed
- ¼ cup fresh mint leaves
- 2 tablespoons freshly squeezed lemon juice
- 8-10 drops liquid stevia
- 1½ cups filtered water
- ½ cup ice cubes

Instructions:

1. Add all ingredients in a high-speed blender and pulse until smooth.
2. Pour the smoothie into 2 serving glasses and serve immediately.

Citrus Apple & Carrot Juice

Yield: 2 servings

Preparation Time: 10 minutes

Total Time: 10 minutes

Ingredients:

- 2 large Granny Smith apples, cored and sliced
- 4 medium carrots, peeled and chopped
- 2 medium grapefruit, peeled and seeded
- 1 teaspoon freshly squeezed lemon juice

Instructions:

1. Add all ingredients in a juicer and extract the juice according to manufacturer's instructions.
2. Transfer into 2 glasses and serve immediately.

Green Veggies & Fruit Juice

Yield: 2 servings

Preparation Time: 10 minutes

Total Time: 10 minutes

Ingredients:

- 2 small green apples, cored and sliced
- 2 small pears, cored and sliced
- 3 cups fresh spinach leaves
- 6 medium celery stalks, chopped
- 1 lemon, peeled and seeded

Instructions:

3. Add all ingredients in a juicer and extract the juice according to manufacturer's instructions.
4. Transfer into 2 glasses and serve immediately.

Orange Juice

Yield: 2 servings

Preparation Time: 10 minutes

Total Time: 10 minutes

Ingredients:

- 8 medium oranges, peeled and sectioned

Instructions:

1. In a juicer, add the orange pieces and extract the juice according to manufacturer's instructions.
2. Transfer into 2 glasses and serve immediately.

Watermelon Juice

Yield: 2 servings

Preparation Time: 10 minutes

Total Time: 10 minutes

Ingredients:

- 4 cups fresh watermelon, seeded and chopped
- Pinch of salt
- Pinch of freshly ground black pepper

Instructions:

1. Add all ingredients in a juicer and extract the juice according to manufacturer's instructions.
2. Transfer into 2 glasses and serve immediately.

Strawberry Juice

Yield: 3 servings

Preparation Time: 10 minutes

Total Time: 10 minutes

Ingredients:

- 2 cups fresh strawberries, hulled and sliced
- 2 cups chilled water
- 1 teaspoon freshly squeezed lime juice
- 1-2 drops liquid stevia

Instructions:

1. In a blender, add all the ingredients and pulse until pureed finely.
2. Through a cheesecloth-lined strainer, strain the juice and transfer into serving glasses.
3. Serve immediately.

Apple, Grapefruit & Carrot Juice

Yield: 2 servings

Preparation Time: 10 minutes

Total Time: 10 minutes

Ingredients:

- 2 large Granny Smith apples, cored and sliced
- 2 medium grapefruits, peeled and seeded
- 4 medium carrots, peeled and chopped
- 1 teaspoon freshly squeezed lemon juice

Instructions:

1. Add all ingredients in a juicer and extract the juice according to manufacturer's instructions.
2. Transfer into 2 glasses and serve immediately.

Apple & Pomegranate Juice

Yield: 2 servings

Preparation Time: 10 minutes

Total Time: 10 minutes

Ingredients:

- 2 cups fresh pomegranate seeds
- 2 large Granny Smith apples, cored and sliced
- 2 teaspoons freshly squeezed lemon juice
- Pinch of freshly ground black pepper

Instructions:

1. Add all ingredients in a juicer and extract the juice according to manufacturer's instructions.
2. Transfer into 2 glasses and serve immediately.

Apple, Beet & Carrot Juice

Yield: 2 servings

Preparation Time: 10 minutes

Total Time: 10 minutes

Ingredients:

- 3 large carrots, peeled and chopped
- 3 medium red beets, trimmed, peeled and chopped
- 1 large Granny Smith apple, cored and sliced
- 1 large green apple, , cored and sliced

Instructions:

1. Add all ingredients in a juicer and extract the juice according to manufacturer's instructions.
2. Transfer into 2 glasses and serve immediately.

Citrus Spinach & Celery Juice

Yield: 2 servings

Preparation Time: 10 minutes

Total Time: 10 minutes

Ingredients:

- 3 cups fresh spinach, chopped
- 2 large celery stalks, chopped
- 2 large green apples, cored and sliced
- 1 large orange, peeled, seeded and sectioned
- 1 tablespoon freshly squeezed lime juice
- 1 tablespoon freshly squeezed lemon juice

Instructions:

1. Add all ingredients in a juicer and extract the juice according to manufacturer's instructions.
2. Transfer into 2 glasses and serve immediately.

Green Veggies Juice

Yield: 2 servings

Preparation Time: 10 minutes

Total Time: 10 minutes

Ingredients:

- 4 small celery stalks
- 3 cups fresh spinach leaves
- 1 cup fresh kale leaves
- 1 (½-inch) piece fresh ginger, peeled
- 1 lime, halved

Instructions:

1. Add all ingredients in a juicer and extract the juice according to manufacturer's instructions.
2. Transfer into 2 glasses and serve immediately.

Chapter 9: Salad Recipes

Strawberry & Spinach Salad

Yield: 4 servings

Preparation Time: 15 minutes

Total Time: 15 minutes

Ingredients:

For Salad:

- 2 cups fresh strawberries, hulled and sliced
- 1½ cups fresh baby spinach
- ¼ cup walnuts, chopped

For Dressing:

- 1 tablespoon balsamic vinegar
- 1 tablespoon freshly squeezed lemon juice
- 1 tablespoon extra-virgin olive oil
- 1-2 drops liquid stevia
- Pinch of sea salt
- Freshly ground black pepper, as required

Instructions:

1. For salad: in a large serving bowl, add the strawberries and spinach and mix.

2. For dressing: in a small bowl, add all the ingredients and beat until well combined.

3. Place the dressing over salad and toss to coat well.

4. Top with walnuts and serve immediately.

Pear & Brussels Sprout Salad

Yield: 4 servings

Preparation Time: 15 minutes

Total Time: 15 minutes

Ingredients:

For Salad:

- 2 large pears, cred and spiralized with Blade C
- 2 cups Brussels sprout, trimmed and sliced thinly
- 4 cups fresh salad greens, chopped finely
- ½ cup almonds, chopped

For Dressing:

- 1 tablespoon shallot, minced
- 3 tablespoons apple cider vinegar
- 3 tablespoons extra-virgin olive oil
- 1 tablespoon pure maple syrup
- 2 teaspoons Dijon mustard
- Freshly ground black pepper, as required

Instructions:

1. For salad: in a large serving bowl, add all the pears, Brussels sprout and salad greens and mix.
2. For dressing: in another bowl, add all the ingredients and beat until well combined.

3. Pour the dressing over salad and toss to coat well.

4. Top with almonds and serve immediately.

Chicken & Strawberry Salad

Yield: 8 servings

Preparation Time: 20 minutes

Cooking Time: 16 minutes

Total Time: 36 minutes

Ingredients:

- 2 pounds boneless, skinless chicken breasts
- 2 tablespoons olive oil
- ¼ cup freshly squeezed lemon juice
- 2 tablespoons granulated Erythritol
- 1 garlic clove, minced
- Salt and freshly ground black pepper, as required
- 4 cups fresh strawberries
- 8 cups fresh spinach, torn

Instructions:

1. For marinade: in a large bowl, add oil, lemon juice, Erythritol, garlic, salt and black pepper and beat until well combined.
2. In a large resealable plastic bag, place the chicken and ¾ cup of marinade.
3. Seal bag and shake to coat well.
4. Refrigerate overnight.

5. Cover the bowl of remaining marinade and refrigerate before serving.

6. Preheat the grill to medium heat. Grease the grill grate.

7. Remove the chicken from bag and discard the marinade.

8. Place the chicken onto grill grate and grill, covered for about 5-8 minutes per side.

9. Remove chicken from grill and cut into bite sized pieces.

10. In a large bowl, add the chicken pieces, strawberries and spinach and mix.

11. Place the reserved marinade and toss to coat.

12. Serve immediately.

Chicken & Avocado Salad

Yield: 4 servings

Preparation Time: 15 minutes

Total Time: 15 minutes

Ingredients:

- 2 large avocados, peeled, pitted and chopped
- ½ cup fresh basil leaves
- 3 tablespoons extra-virgin olive oil
- Salt and freshly ground black pepper, as required
- 4 (4-ounce) cooked chicken breasts, shredded
- ¼ cup cashews

Instructions:

- Add all ingredients except chicken in a food processor and cashews and pulse until smooth.
- In a bowl, add chicken and avocado mixture and gently, toss to coat.
- Top with cashews and serve immediately.

Steak & Plum Salad

Yield: 4 servings

Preparation Time: 15 minutes

Cooking Time: 12 minutes

Total Time: 27 minutes

Ingredients:

- 4 teaspoons freshly squeezed lemon juice, divided
- 1½ tablespoons extra-virgin olive oil, divided
- Sea salt and freshly ground black pepper, as required
- 1 pound flank steak, trimmed
- Olive oil cooking spray
- 1 teaspoon raw honey
- 8 cups fresh baby arugula
- 3 plums, pitted and sliced thinly
- ¼ cup feta cheese, crumbled

Instructions:

1. In a large bowl, add 1 teaspoon of lemon juice, 1½ teaspoons of extra-virgin olive oil, salt and black pepper and mix until well combined.
2. Add the steak and coat with mixture generously.
3. Grease a non-stick skillet with a little cooking spray and heat over medium-high heat.
4. Add the steak and cook for about 5-6 minutes per side.

5. Transfer the steak onto a cutting board and set aside for about 10 minutes before slicing.

6. With a sharp knife, cut the beef steak diagonally across grain in desired size slices.

7. In a large bowl, add the remaining lemon juice, oil, honey, sea salt and black pepper and beat until well combined.

8. Add the arugula and toss to coat well.

9. Divide the arugula onto 4 serving plates.

10. Top with beef slices, plum slices and cheese evenly and serve.

Salmon Salad

Yield: 4 servings

Preparation Time: 20 minutes

Cooking Time: 15 minutes

Total Time: 35 minutes

Ingredients:

- 2 (6-ounce) salmon fillets
- 4 tablespoons olive oil, divided
- Sea salt and freshly ground black pepper, as required
- 4 ounce fresh mushrooms (of your choice), sliced
- 1 avocado, peeled, pitted and cubed
- 12 grape tomatoes, halved
- 8 ounces lettuce, torn
- ¼ cup fresh cilantro, chopped
- 2 tablespoons balsamic vinegar

Instructions:

1. Preheat the broiler of oven.
2. Line a large baking sheet with a piece of foil.
3. Coat the salmon fillets with 1 tablespoon of oil and sprinkle with salt and black pepper.
4. Arrange the salmon fillets onto the prepared baking sheet in a single layer.
5. Broil for about 15 minutes.

6. Remove from the oven an place the salmon fillets onto a cutting board for about 5 minutes before cutting.

7. With a sharp knife, cut the salmon in bite sized pieces.

8. Meanwhile, in a skillet, heat 1 tablespoon of the oil over medium heat and sauté the mushrooms for about 6-8 minutes.

9. Remove the pan from heat and set aside to cool slightly.

10. In a large bowl, add the salmon, mushrooms and remaining all ingredients and toss to coat well.

11. Serve immediately.

Shrimp, Apple & Carrot Salad

Yield: 4 servings

Preparation Time: 20 minutes

Cooking Time: 3 minutes

Total Time: 23 minutes

Ingredients:

- 12 medium shrimp
- 1½ cups Granny Smith apple, cored and sliced thinly
- 1½ cups carrot, peeled and cut into matchsticks
- ½ cup fresh mint leaves, chopped
- 2 tablespoons balsamic vinegar
- ¼ cup extra-virgin olive oil
- 1 teaspoon lemongrass, chopped
- 1 teaspoon garlic, minced
- 2 sprigs fresh cilantro, leaves separated and chopped

Instructions:

1. In a large pan of the salted boiling water, add the shrimp and lemon and cook for about 3 minutes.
2. Remove the pan from heat and drain the shrimp well.
3. Set aside to cool.
4. After cooling, peel and devein the shrimps.
5. Transfer the shrimp into a large bowl.

6. Add the remaining all ingredients except cilantro and gently, stir to combine.
7. Cover the bowl and refrigerate for about 1 hour.
8. Top with cilantro just before serving.

Shrimp & Greens Salad

Yield: 6 servings

Preparation Time: 15 minutes

Cooking Time: 6 minutes

Total Time: 21 minutes

Ingredients:

- 1 tablespoon olive oil
- 1 garlic clove, crushed and divided
- 2 tablespoons fresh rosemary, chopped
- 1 pound shrimp, peeled and deveined
- Sea salt and freshly ground black pepper, as required
- 4 cups fresh arugula
- 2 cups Romaine lettuce, torn
- 2 tablespoons olive oil
- 2 tablespoons freshly squeezed lime juice

Instructions:

1. In a large skillet, melt the oil over medium heat and sauté 1 garlic clove for about 1 minute.
2. Add the shrimp with salt and black pepper and cook for about 4-5 minutes.
3. Remove the pan from heat and set aside to cool.
4. Ina large bowl, add the shrimp, arugula, lettuce, oil, lime juice, salt and black pepper and gently, toss to coat.

5. Serve immediately.

Black Beans & Corn Salad

Yield: 6 servings

Preparation Time: 15 minutes

Total Time: 15 minutes

Ingredients:

- 2 (16-ounce) cans black beans, drained and rinsed
- 1 cup whole corn kernel
- ¼ cup fresh parsley, chopped
- 2 tablespoon red onion, minced
- ¼ cup balsamic vinegar
- 2 tablespoons olive oil
- 1 teaspoon freshly squeezed lemon juice
- 1 teaspoon garlic, minced
- 1 teaspoon honey
- Freshly ground black pepper, as required

Instructions:

1. For salad: in a large serving bowl, add the black beans, corn, red onion and parsley and mix well.
2. For dressing: in another bowl, add the vinegar, olive oil, lemon juice, garlic, honey and black pepper and beat until well combined.
3. Pour the dressing over salad and gently, toss to coat well.

4. Refrigerate the salad for at least 30 minutes before
    serving.

Quinoa Salad

Yield: 3 servings

Preparation Time: 20 minutes

Cooking Time: 20 minutes

Total Time: 40 minutes

Ingredients:

For Quinoa:

- 1 teaspoon olive oil
- 1 cup golden quinoa, rinsed and drained
- 1¾ cups filtered water

For Salad:

- 2 medium seedless cucumbers, chopped
- 8 small red radishes, trimmed and chopped
- 1 large red onion, chopped
- ¼ cup almonds, chopped
- 1 avocado, peeled, pitted and chopped

For Vinaigrette:

- 1 tablespoon fresh dill, minced
- 1 teaspoon fresh lemon zest, grated finely
- 3 tablespoons extra-virgin olive oil
- 2 tablespoons freshly squeezed lemon juice
- ½ tablespoon balsamic vinegar

- Freshly ground black pepper, as required

Instructions:

1. For quinoa: in a pan, heat the oil over medium-high heat and cook the quinoa for about 1 minute, stirring continuously.
2. Add the water and bring to a boil.
3. Decrease the heat to low and simmer, covered for about 15-20 minutes or until all the liquid is absorbed.
4. Remove from heat and set the pan aside, covered for about 5 minutes.
5. Uncover and with a fork, fluff the quinoa.
6. Transfer the quinoa into a large bowl and set aside to cool completely.
7. In the bowl of quinoa, add all salad ingredients except avocado.
8. For vinaigrette: in another bowl, add all the ingredients and beat until well combined.
9. Pour the vinaigrette over salad and gently, toss to coat well.
10. Serve with the topping of avocado.

Chapter 10: Soup Recipes

Tomato Soup

Yield: 4 servings

Preparation Time: 10 minutes

Cooking Time: 20 minutes

Total Time: 30 minutes

Ingredients:

- 2 tablespoons olive oil
- 1 cup red onion, chopped
- 2¼ cups fresh tomatoes, chopped finely
- ½ teaspoon dried thyme, crushed
- 3 cups filtered water
- ¼ cup fresh basil leaves, chopped
- Salt and freshly ground black pepper, as required

Instructions:

1. Heat the oil in a large soup pan over medium heat and sauté onion for about 4-5 minutes.
2. Add the tomatoes, thyme and water and bring to a boil.
3. Decrease the heat to low and simmer, covered for about 15 minutes.
4. Remove the soup pan from heat and set aside to cool slightly.

5. In a blender, add soup in batches and pulse until smooth.

6. Return the soup in the same pan over medium heat.

7. Stir in basil and cook for about 3-4 minutes.

8. Season with salt and black pepper and serve hot.

Collard Greens Soup

Yield: 6 servings

Preparation Time: 15 minutes

Cooking Time: 50 minutes

Total Time: 1 hour 5 minutes

Ingredients:

- 2 tablespoons olive oil
- 1 large white onion, chopped
- Pinch of salt
- 2 large leeks, sliced
- 2 tablespoons fresh ginger, minced
- 1 large bunch collard greens, chopped
- 8 cups low-fat chicken broth
- Freshly ground black pepper, as required
- 1 tablespoon freshly squeezed lemon juice

Instructions:

1. Heat the oil in a large soup pan over low heat and cook the onion and salt for about 20 minutes, stirring occasionally.
2. Stir in the leeks and cook for about 10 minutes.
3. Stir in ginger and greens and cook for about 5 minutes.
4. Add the broth and stir to combine.
5. Increase the heat to medium-high and bring to a boil.

6. Decrease the heat to medium and cook for about 10 minutes.

7. Remove the soup pan from heat and set aside to cool slightly.

8. In a blender, add the soup mixture and pulse until smooth.

9. Return the soup in the same pan over medium heat and cook for about 5 minutes.

10. Stir in the lemon juice and black pepper and serve hot.

Yellow Squash Soup

Yield: 6 servings

Preparation Time: 15 minutes

Cooking Time: 35 minutes

Total Time: 50 minutes

Ingredients:

- 2 tablespoons olive oil
- 2 small yellow onions, chopped
- 6 garlic cloves, minced
- 6 cups yellow squash, cubed
- 2 fresh thyme sprigs
- 2 fresh rosemary sprigs
- 4 cups low-fat vegetable broth
- ¼ teaspoon cayenne pepper
- Freshly ground black pepper, as required
- 2 tablespoons freshly squeezed lemon juice
- 2 teaspoons fresh lemon peel, grated finely

Instructions:

1. Heat the oil in a large soup pan over medium heat and sauté the onions for about 5-6 minutes.
2. Add in the garlic and sauté for about 1 minute.
3. Add the yellow squash cubes and cook for about 5 minutes, stirring occasionally.

4. Stir in the thyme, rosemary, broth, cayenne pepper and black pepper and bring to a boil.

5. Decrease the heat to low and cook, covered for about 15-20 minutes.

6. Remove from the heat and discard the herb sprigs.

7. Remove the soup pan from heat and set aside to cool slightly.

8. In a large blender, add the soup in 2 batches and pulse until smooth.

9. Return the soup into the same pan over medium heat.

10. Stir in the lemon juice and cook for about 2-3 minutes or until heated completely.

11. Remove from the heat and serve hot with the garnishing of lemon peel.

Zucchini Soup

Yield: 3 servings

Preparation Time: 15 minutes

Cooking Time: 30 minutes

Total Time: 45 minutes

Ingredients:

- 1 large shallot, chopped roughly
- 1 jalapeño pepper, seeded and chopped
- 1 garlic clove, peeled
- 2 teaspoons olive oil
- 3 medium zucchinis, chopped
- 2 cups low-fat chicken broth
- 2 tablespoons fresh dill, chopped
- ½ cup fat-free plain Greek yogurt
- Freshly ground black pepper, as required
- 2 tablespoons fresh parsley, chopped

Instructions:

1. In a food processor, add the shallot, jalapeno and garlic and pulse until finely chopped.
2. Heat the oil in a large soup pan over medium heat and sauté the shallot mixture for about 3-5 minutes.
3. Add the zucchini and broth and stir to combine.
4. Simmer for about 15-20 minutes.

5. Remove the soup pan from heat and discard the herb sprigs.

6. Set the pan aside to cool slightly.

7. In a large blender, add the soup and yogurt in 2 batches and pulse until smooth.

8. Return the soup into the same pan over medium heat.

9. Stir in the black pepper and cook for about 2-3 minutes or until heated completely.

10. Remove from the heat and serve hot with the garnishing of parsley.

Broccoli & Avocado Soup

Yield: 5 servings

Preparation Time: 15 minutes

Cooking Time: 55 minutes

Total Time: 1 hour 10 minutes

Ingredients:

- 2 tablespoons olive oil
- ½ cup yellow onion, chopped
- 1 large garlic clove, minced
- 1 tablespoon fresh thyme, chopped
- ¼ teaspoon ground cumin
- ¼ teaspoon red pepper flakes, crushed
- 2 medium heads broccoli, cut into florets
- 4 cups low-fat vegetable broth
- Freshly ground black pepper, as required
- 1 avocado, peeled, pitted and chopped
- 1 teaspoon fresh cilantro leaves
- 1 teaspoon fresh mint leaves
- 1 tablespoon freshly squeezed lemon juice
- 1 teaspoon pumpkin seeds

Instructions:

1. Heat the oil in a large soup pan over medium heat and sauté the onion for about 4-5 minutes.

2. Add the garlic, thyme, cumin and red pepper flakes and sauté for about 1 minute more.

3. Stir in the broccoli and cook for about 3-4 minutes, stirring frequently.

4. Add the broth and black pepper and stir to combine.

5. Increase the heat to high and bring to a boil.

6. Decrease the heat to medium-low and simmer, covered for about 30-35 minutes.

7. Remove the soup pan from heat and set aside to cool slightly.

8. In a high-speed blender, place the soup mixture, avocado, cilantro and mint in 2 batches and pulse until smooth.

9. Return the soup into the same pan over medium-low heat and cook for about 3-5 minutes or until heated completely.

10. Stir in the lemon juice, salt and black pepper and remove from the heat.

11. Serve hot with the topping of pumpkin seeds.

Cauliflower & Ginger Soup

Yield: 2 servings

Preparation Time: 15 minutes

Cooking Time: 50 minutes

Total Time: 1 hour 5 minutes

Ingredients:

- 2 teaspoons olive oil
- ½ cup yellow onion, chopped
- 1 large head cauliflower, cut into small florets
- 1 (1-inch) piece fresh ginger, chopped
- Freshly ground black pepper, as required
- 3 cups low-fat chicken broth

Instructions:

1. In a large soup pan, heat oil over medium heat and sauté the onion for about 1 minute.
2. Add the cauliflower and cook, covered for about 10 minutes, stirring occasionally.
3. Add the remaining ingredients and bring to a boil
4. Decrease the heat to low and simmer, covered for about 30 minutes.
5. Remove the soup pan from heat and set aside to cool slightly.

6. In a blender, add the soup mixture in 2 batches and pulse until smooth.

7. Return the soup in the same pan over medium-low heat and simmer for about 4-5 minutes or until heated completely.

8. Serve hot.

Carrot & Ginger Soup

Yield: 4 servings

Preparation Time: 15 minutes

Cooking Time: 30 minutes

Total Time: 45 minutes

Ingredients:

- 1 tablespoon olive oil
- 1 medium brown onion chopped
- 2 garlic cloves, minced
- 1 long red chili, chopped
- 1 (¼-inch) piece fresh turmeric, peeled and sliced
- 1 (½-inch) piece fresh galangal, peeled and sliced
- 1 (1-inch) piece fresh ginger, peeled and sliced
- 4 cups carrots, peeled and chopped
- 2 lemongrass stalks
- 2 cups water
- 2 cups low-fat vegetable broth
- Freshly ground black pepper, as required
- 2 tablespoons fresh cilantro, chopped

Instructions:

1. Heat the oil in a large soup pan over medium heat and sauté the onion for about 5 minutes.

2. Add the garlic, red chili, turmeric, galangal and ginger and sauté for about 5 minutes.

3. Add the carrots, lemongrass stalks, water and broth and bring to a boil.

4. Decrease the heat to low and simmer for about 15-20 minutes.

1. Remove the soup pan from heat and set aside to cool slightly.

2. Discard the lemongrass stalks.

3. In a blender, add the soup in 2 batches and pulse until smooth.

4. Return the soup in the same pan over medium-low heat and simmer for about 4-5 minutes or until heated completely.

5. Stir in the black pepper and remove from the heat.

6. Serve hot with the garnishing of cilantro.

Sweet Potato & Bell Pepper Soup

Yield: 4 servings

Preparation Time: 15 minutes

Cooking Time: 30 minutes

Total Time: 45 minutes

Ingredients:

- 2 tablespoons olive oil
- 1 medium white onion, chopped
- 1 red bell pepper, seeded and chopped
- 2 garlic cloves, minced
- 1 (1-inch) piece fresh ginger, grated
- 1 teaspoon dried rosemary, crushed
- 1 teaspoon dried thyme, crushed
- 1 teaspoon ground cinnamon
- ½ teaspoon cayenne pepper
- ½ cup tomato puree
- 1 tablespoon maple syrup
- 3 cups low-fat vegetable broth
- 2 large sweet potatoes, peeled and chopped
- 2 tablespoons freshly squeezed lemon juice
- Freshly ground black pepper, as required
- ¼ cup fresh cilantro, chopped

Instructions:

1. Heat the oil in a large soup pan over medium heat and sauté the onion for about 5 minutes.
2. Add the bell pepper, garlic, ginger, dried herbs, cinnamon and cayenne pepper and sauté for about 1 minute.
3. Stir in the tomato puree and maple syrup and cook for about 1 minute.
4. Stir in the sweet potatoes and broth and bring to a boil.
5. Simmer for about 10-15 minutes, stirring occasionally.
6. Remove the soup pan from heat and set aside to cool slightly.
7. In a blender, add the soup in 2 batches and pulse until smooth.
8. Return the soup in the same pan over medium-low heat and simmer for about 4-5 minutes or until heated completely.
9. Stir in the lemon juice and black pepper and remove from the heat.
10. Serve hot with the garnishing of cilantro.

Butternut Squash & Pear Soup

Yield: 3 servings

Preparation Time: 15 minutes

Cooking Time: 38 minutes

Total Time: 53 minutes

Ingredients:

- 1 tablespoon olive oil
- 1 medium yellow onion, chopped
- 1 garlic clove, minced
- 1 teaspoon fresh ginger, minced
- 2 pears, peeled, cored and chopped
- 1½ pound butternut squash, peeled, seeded and chopped
- 4 cups low-fat vegetable broth
- ¼ cup unsweetened almond milk
- Pinch of freshly ground black pepper
- 2 tablespoons fresh basil leaves, chopped

Instructions:

1. Heat the oil in a large soup pan over medium heat and sauté the onion for about 3-4 minutes.
2. Add the garlic and ginger and sauté for about 1 minute.
3. Add the pears, squash and broth and stir to combine.
4. Increase the heat to high and bring to a boil.

5. Decrease the heat to medium-low and simmer, covered for about 20-25 minutes.
6. Stir in the almond milk and cook for about 5 minutes.
7. Stir in the black pepper and remove from heat.
8. Remove the soup pan from heat and set aside to cool slightly.
9. Transfer the soup mixture in a blender in batches and pulse until smooth.
10. Return the soup in the same pan over medium heat and cook for 2-3 minutes or until heated completely.
11. Serve hot with the garnishing of basil leaves.

Pumpkin & Black Beans Soup

Yield: 6 servings

Preparation Time: 15 minutes

Cooking Time: 35 minutes

Total Time: 50 minutes

Ingredients:

- 2 tablespoons olive oil
- 1 medium white onion, chopped
- 4 garlic cloves, minced
- 1 tablespoon ground cumin
- 1 teaspoon red chili powder
- Freshly ground black pepper, as required
- 2 (15-ounce) cans black beans, rinsed and drained
- 1 (16-ounce) can sugar-free pumpkin puree
- 1 cup fresh tomatoes, chopped finely
- 2 cups low-fat chicken broth
- ¼ cup fat-free plain Greek yogurt
- ¼ cup fresh cilantro, chopped

Instructions:

1. Heat the oil in a large soup pan over medium heat and sauté the onion for about 4-5 minutes.
2. Add the garlic, cumin, chili powder and black pepper and sauté for about 1 minute.

3. Add the black beans, pumpkin, tomatoes and broth and stir to combine.

4. Increase the heat to medium-high and bring to a boil.

5. Decrease the heat and simmer, uncovered for about 25 minutes, stirring occasionally.

6. Remove from the heat and stir in the yogurt.

7. With an immersion blender, blend the soup until smooth.

8. Serve hot with the garnishing of cilantro.

Chapter 11: Tips for Dating Out

It is true that your life will not remain the same after this weight loss gastric sleeve surgery. Every time you will go out, you can't simply eat everything on the menu. A dieter must consider the following points in mind before placing the order:

1. Order small portions
2. Eat slowly and chew properly
3. Do not order bread and butter for the table
4. Avoid fried food and order boiled, steamed, or grilled food instead.
5. Do not order drinks along with the meal.
6. Order soft desserts like pudding and ice creams.
7. Do not order food like steaks, bread, or asparagus that are difficult to chew completely.

Chapter 12: Conclusion

Perhaps, weight loss can be achieved when we provide the body just enough calories to meet the nutritional needs and nothing more than that. The caloric restriction can be maintained by controlling the dietary patterns or reducing the amount of food intake. There are people who simply cannot afford to make the dietary changes, so they can take benefit from gastric sleeve surgery to reduce daily food consumption and achieve weight loss in no time. The gastric sleeve surgery changes a person's life altogether. Therefore, it requires a special diet to support the changes. In this cook, we have shared all the suitable bariatric diet recipes, to make it easier for those who are going through post-op complications.